Y0-AGK-424

The Origin and Diversification of Language

Editors

Nina G. Jablonski
California Academy of Sciences, San Francisco, California

Leslie C. Aiello
University College London, London, England

with the editorial assistance of Nancy Gee

Wattis Symposium Series in Anthropology

MEMOIRS OF THE CALIFORNIA ACADEMY OF SCIENCES
Number 24

San Francisco, California
July 17, 1998

SCIENTIFIC PUBLICATION COMMITTEE:

Alan E. Leviton, *Editor*
Katie Martin, *Managing Editor*

©1998 by the California Academy of Sciences
Golden Gate Park
San Francisco, California 94118

Library of Congress Catalog Card Number: 98-71454

ISBN 0-940228-44-0 (cloth)
ISBN 0-040228-46-7 (paper)

Printed in the United States of America by the Allen Press

Distributed by the University of California Press

Wattis Symposium Series in Anthropology

MEMOIRS OF THE CALIFORNIA ACADEMY
OF SCIENCES, NUMBER 24

The Origin and Diversification of Language

TABLE OF CONTENTS

Preface

Since the beginnings of humankind, there has been no greater innovation than language. The signal importance of language in human evolution has long been appreciated, but until recently the tools available for study of the origin and diversification of language were limited to relatively simple comparative anatomical and linguistic studies, and to studies of language acquisition in apes. The study of the origin and diversification of language today benefits from advances in those areas plus many others, from neurobiology and molecular biology, to cognitive and developmental psychology, to animal behavior, archaeology and historical linguistics.

This short volume represents the edited and peer-reviewed proceedings of the Third Wattis Symposium in Anthropology, on the Origin and Diversification of Language, held at the California Academy of Sciences on 12 April 1997. Like the previous two Wattis Symposia, the aim of the Third was to address a topic of broad interest in anthropology, the illumination of which would benefit from the contributions of workers from many disciplines. While many approaches could have been taken in the organization of the symposium and this volume, coverage of some of the startling advances made in recent years in the study of the biological underpinnings of language was deemed of high priority. The first half of this book is, thus, devoted to explorations of the similarities and differences between animal communication and human language (Marler), the anatomical foundations of languages (Aiello and R.D. Martin), and the functional neuroanatomy of the organization of semantic knowledge in the brain (A. Martin). In the latter half of the book the archaeological evidence for the origin of language is explored (Mellars), followed by an examination of language as an adaptation in the evolutionary sense (Pinker). The book is rounded out by two chapters on the diversification of languages, one from the point of view of the archaeological record (Renfrew), one from that of historical linguistics (Nichols). This is intended as a provocative, not a comprehensive, collection of studies of language origin and diversification, and one ideally suited for advanced undergraduate or graduate students eager to learn of the present and emerging controversies in this important field.

The Third Wattis Symposium in Anthropology and this volume would not have been possible without the support of many devoted individuals. Mrs. Phyllis Wattis herself deserves greatest thanks for her continued generous financial support and her inspiring enthusiasm, which seems only to increase from one symposium to another. Within the California Academy of Sciences itself, Nancy Gee of the Department of Anthropology is thanked for the work she contributed toward the organization of the symposium, but most especially for her painstaking work in typesetting this volume.

Nina G. Jablonski
Irvine Chair and Curator of Anthropology
California Academy of Sciences
23 March 1998

Animal Communication and Human Language

Peter Marler
Center for Animal Behavior
University of California
Davis, CA 95616

A reductionistic approach is taken to some similarities and contrasts between language and the natural communicative behavior of animals, especially vocalizations of birds and nonhuman primates. Three basic questions are addressed: 1) What do animal sounds mean; 2) Do animals "intend" to communicate; and 3) Do animals speak in sentences? Using as a point of departure the widespread view that animal sounds are all nonsymbolic displays of emotion, a case is made that the alarm signals and food calls of some animals are indeed symbolic. They function referentially in the sense that they "stand for" something specific in the environment such as food or a particular predator. The presence or absence of a potential "audience" for their calls affects the readiness of animals to give alarm signals when they sight a predator, or food calls when they discover something edible, as would be expected if they "intend" to communicate. Some animals, like humans, have vocalizations that are learned, and passed by tradition from generation to generation. But only humans have the capacity to recombine them into sentences. It is true that certain animals, especially songbirds, can recombine learned sounds into many different sequences, thus creating large signal repertoires. The sequences are not sentences, however, but affective, nonsymbolic songs, more like music than language.

Anyone who ventures to speculate about the relationship between animal communication and language is confronted by obstacles on all sides. How should the comparison be conducted? We are a single species. Animals are legion, and each has its own way of communicating, some completely alien to us. What should we compare? Only by the most indirect means can we gain access to the mysteries of the electrical senses of fish, the substrate vibrations that frogs and many insects use to talk to one another, the ultrasonic signals of bats and rodents, or the infrasound of elephants. The most ubiquitous medium of all for biological communication, the sense of smell, is one that many of us choose to mask or ignore. Whenever living things of any species gather together, more often than not they eventually communicate, the leading subject is usually sex, and the primary vehicles will be, not sounds, but pheromones, perhaps sometimes more important in our own lives than we acknowledge.

The Origin and Diversification of Language
Editors, N.G. Jablonski & L.C. Aiello

Memoirs of the California Academy of Sciences
Number 24, Copyright ©1998

Comparisons of the intricacies of visual communication, both paralinguistic and linguistic, including signing and facial expressions, in animals and in humans, would surely be illuminating (*cf.* Marler & Evans 1997). But if the subject is commonalties and contrasts with language, communication by ear has to be the primary focus.

Then there are other problems. We are born and bred as users of language. From birth, and perhaps even in the womb, we bring to bear every physiological, behavioral and cognitive specialization we possess, as we develop our uniquely human system of language and thought. As insiders we have a privileged, intimate view of the almost unlimited potential of language, and our insights are authentic to a degree that we can never hope to attain with the communication systems of other species. By comparison with language studies, in all of their many guises, investigations of animal communication are still in their infancy. If we are ever to make any scientific progress, our present state of relative ignorance almost forces us to simplify, and focus, not on the highest achievements, but on the fundamental principles that underlie communication in animals. It is in this reductionistic spirit that I pose three basic questions, drawing illustrations from the animal vocal communication systems of the animals that I know best, namely birds and monkeys. The first question is what do animal sounds mean, if anything at all? Are they just displays of emotion, or is there reason to believe that some of their calls serve as symbols? Secondly, do we have any indications that animals intend to communicate rather than simply signaling reflexively? Finally and most importantly, I will grapple with one aspect of the great linguistic theme that we identify especially with the work of Noam Chomsky, the question of syntax. Adopting once more a reductionistic approach, I will pose the question: Do animals speak in sentences? In what follows I shall discuss only the natural communicative behavior of animals. I shall not consider any of the studies in which humans have taught animals to perform somewhat human-like behavior, using signing, sounds or other tokens as vehicles for communicating with their trainer. In such studies it is not easy to determine how much of the behavior comes naturally, and how much is inculcated by the experimenter.

What Do Animal Sounds Mean?

The thinking of zoologists about the semantics of natural animal calls, especially the calls of nonhuman primates, has undergone something of a revolution in the past couple of decades. Not so long ago, speculations about how best to interpret the calls of monkeys were all based on what Donald Griffin (1992) aptly described as the "groans of pain" (GOP) concept of animal communication. The universal assumption underlying the GOP model is that vocalizations of monkeys and other animals are displays of emotion or affect, much like our own facial expressions. Only humans are thought to have progressed beyond this condition, and to have achieved symbolic signaling. Premack (1975:593) stated the prevailing view clearly and succinctly: "Man has both affective and symbolic communication. All other species, except when tutored by man, have only the affective form." According to this view, symbolic signals are presumably those that have identifiable referents in the organism's environment to which the signal can be said to refer, in an abstract, noniconic fashion. For an animal communication system to qualify as symbolic, information about one or more external referents has to be both encoded by signalers and decoded by receivers.

Premack's is not an idiosyncratic view. Affective or emotional signaling is presumed to be a more basic and primitive communicative mode, and as such is a critical antithesis to the kind of symbolic functioning that epitomizes language. This view recurs repeatedly in the literature of many disciplines (Table 1). The underlying logic is often not made fully explicit, however, complicating the task of generalizing from humans to animals, and making it more difficult to decide whether the affective/symbolic dichotomy does in fact provide a useful basis for comparing animal and human communication. Because it is so widespread, I have taken it as one point of departure in analyzing the communicative behavior of animals. There are others, such as semiotic theory, that may prove to be more illuminating in the long run (*e.g.*, Marler 1961, 1992), making use of basic distinctions between signals as icons, indexical signs and symbols (Sebeok 1976). For present purposes, borrowing and adapting from Morris (1946), Cherry (1957), and Zivin (1985), I shall use the term "symbol" to refer to noniconic signals that stand for or represent a referent that is external to the organism, either currently or from memory, and can be interpreted as such by another organism. This usage is somewhat different from that of Smith (1981) who defines a referent as "anything that becomes knowable or predictable through the performance of a signal," presumably whether external or internal. However I shall take the position that a symbol cannot refer to itself. Thus, a sign or manifestation of an internal state, such as a motivational or emotional condition, cannot symbolize itself. It is rather an index of that state. An internal state can, however, mediate in the production of a symbol with a set of external objects and events as its referents if experience of those referents or "designate" reliably engenders that state. Signals that lack the property of symbolization of external referent I shall call simply nonsymbolic signals. Expressions of emotion are viewed by many as falling into this category (Table 1), although, as I will show, it can be argued that this is not always true.

If we accept that, by definition, affective signals have no clear or specific symbolic referents, emotion-based calls are surely widespread in animals, and perhaps

TABLE 1. Interpretations of animal signals as manifestations of affect, emotion, or motivation: Statements from a variety of sources about the meaning of animal signals, especially monkey calls.

A. "The noises made by monkeys express their mood, and are effective in communicating it to others." (Rowell & Hinde 1962:279, zoologists).

B. "Nonhuman primates can send complex messages about their motivational states; they communicate almost nothing about the state of their physical environments." (Lancaster 1965:64, anthropologist).

C. "All signals (of animals) appear to be clearly related to the immediate emotional states of the signaling individuals and their levels of arousal." (Bastian 1965:598, linguist).

D. "The use of both the face and the voice by rhesus monkeys in their natural habitat seems to be restricted to circumstances that connote emotion." (Myers 1976:747-748, neurobiologist).

E. "The nonhuman primate does not use the auditory medium to communicate whatever conceptual knowledge it possesses. The vocal repertoire appears to relate to affective rather than cognitive dimensions, the nature of the signal reflecting the emotional disposition of the caller." (Marin *et al.* 1979:184, psychiatrists).

F. "The signal emitted by an animal is an expression of its affective condition, and the reception of the signal indicates the infection of others by the same condition — nothing more." (Luria 1982:29, psychologist).

G. "Man has both affective and symbolic communication. All other species, except when tutored by man, have only the affective form." (Premack 1975:593, psychologist).

even the rule. But there are others that do not fit neatly into the GOP mold. A few years ago the revisionist process began in earnest with descriptive studies of the remarkably rich repertoire of alarm calls of the vervet monkey in Africa by Struhsaker (1967). Seyfarth, Cheney and Marler (1980a, b) took the further step of playing tape-recordings of alarm calls to free-ranging monkeys. Vervet monkeys live, not like most of its dozen or so congeners, in the depths of the African rain forest, but on the forest edge. They often venture out on to the savannah, where they are exposed to many predators, hence perhaps the enrichment of their alarm call repertoire. Different predators call for different escape strategies and distinct alarm calls aid them in deciding which strategy to adopt. Some vervet alarm calls are quite general, simply leading companions to become more vigilant, but other calls are so specific that it is not unreasonable to think of them as labels or names, such as the leopard call, the snake call, or the eagle call. This viewpoint seemed all the more reasonable after a long series of playbacks of tape recordings had been conducted in the absence of any predators in their natural habitat, in the African bush, at Amboseli, in Kenya. The calls elicited those natural reactions that were already known to be specific and appropriate to the particular predator. They differed in ways that made good ecological sense, given the different hunting strategies of these predators. The monkeys searched the sky and ran into bushes in response to eagle calls, leaped up into the canopy of fever trees in response to leopard calls, and reared up on their hind legs and scanned the underbrush when a snake call was played. In other words, there was every indication that, in a formalistic sense, the calls served as symbols for the predators.

Inspired by this new point of view on what animal calls mean, especially as it was developed at length by Cheney and Seyfarth (1981, 1985, 1988, 1990), there have been many other demonstrations of animal alarm calls that display what came to be defined as "functional reference" (Marler, Evans & Hauser 1992; Evans & Marler 1995). The calls function as though they "stand for" the object or "referent" that they represent. In other words, they function as abstract "symbols." They are also "non-iconic" in the sense that their acoustic structure has an arbitrary relationship with the physical features of the referent. To model what seems to be taking place, we have to postulate a formal series of translations or transformations from between (a) the predator, (b) the caller's perception and identification of the predator, (c) production of the appropriate call, and (d) the response that another monkey gives when the call is heard. The question remains, what is really going on in the monkeys' heads? Are they cogitating, or acting reflexively and unconsciously? From one point of view, a cognitive interpretation of this behavioral sequence seems natural. But in the absence of detailed experiments, and without the benefits of introspection, we have no way of knowing whether the transformations that go on in a vervet's head when it hears and responds to another's alarm call involve cognition, conscious or otherwise, or whether they are reflexive, and perhaps even innate, and thus quite un-language like. Yet the alarm calls clearly function referentially, as symbols for both callers and listeners. It is to capture this concept that the term "functional reference" was coined, permitting the issue of reference to be discussed while remaining agnostic on the nature of the underlying mental and neural processes.

In addition to alarm calls, some animals also give food calls (Table 2). In both primates and birds there are now enough well-documented accounts that we can assume that functionally referential food calls are not uncommon in higher vertebrates, conveying as they seem to, not just that food has been found, but with some inkling, understood by others, as to the quality and quantity of the food as well (*e.g.*, Marler *et al.*

TABLE 2. Bird and mammal calls with "meaning": A sampling of some bird and mammal calls that function symbolically.

red jungle fowl	alarm calls food calls	Collias 1987
chickens	alarm calls food calls	Gyger *et al.* 1987 Evans *et al.* 1993 Evans & Marler 1994
lapwings (3 spp)	alarm calls	Walters 1990
chaffinches	alarm calls	Marler 1959b
chimpanzees	food calls	Hauser *et al.* 1993
rhesus macaques	food calls	Hauser & Marler 1993a, b
toque macaques	food calls	Dittus 1984
vervet monkeys	alarm calls	Seyfarth *et al.* 1980
diana monkeys	alarm calls	Zuberbuhler *et al. 1997*
tamarins	food calls	Benz 1993 Benz *et al.* 1992
ring-tailed lemurs	alarm calls	Macedonia 1990
Malaysian tree squirrels (3 spp)	alarm calls	Tamura & Yong 1993
alpine marmots	alarm calls	Boero 1992

1986a; Elowson *et al.* 1991; review in Hauser 1996). Food calling is especially widespread in gallinaceous birds such as pheasants, quail and chickens (*e.g.*, Collias 1960, 1987), studies of which have provided some evidence of deceptive use of food calls to attract others when in fact no food is present (Gyger & Marler 1988). Whether the deception is intentional or the manifestation of a learned habit is moot, and since the subjects in these studies were not monkeys but chickens, most observers display a chauvinistic reluctance to entertain cognitive interpretations of the behavior of a creature as lowly as domestic fowl.

Aside from the slippery issue of deception, studies of these cases of referential alarm and food calls seem to indicate that the GOP point of view is not tenable, assuming that is, that we accept the widespread view that displays of emotion do not have symbolic meanings in the usual sense. This is, in fact, a matter for debate. The key point may be, not that emotional displays are completely lacking in semantic meaning, but rather that there is a difference in the kinds of meanings they encode, perhaps more generalized and unspecified than those we tend to view as diagnostic of language. When a person responds to situations they encounter with either a grunt of rage or a cry of fear we can be fairly sure that the external situations they have encountered are different and we might hazard a guess as to their nature, but at best only in very general terms. A wide range of situations can result in production of the very same angry grunt. Nevertheless the entire set of situations that merit an angry grunt, if we could even characterize it, would be different from the equivalent sets for cries of fear or chuckles of pleasure. So there may be some degree of referentiality less specific than in emotional displays, but this will typically be much less specific than is achievable in language. This relative lack of specificity, compared with what we can accomplish with language, may be one factor that gives rise to the judgment shared by many (Table 1) that there is little common ground between emotional and symbolic behavior. On this basis we may conclude that these cases of highly specific functional reference in animal communication provide some indication of a language-like attribute, but several issues remain equivocal.

We have only limited information on the role of experience in the development of functionally referential communication, an issue that is critical if we are to understand the role of cognition. Learning does seem to play a role in both linking calling to appropriate external stimuli and in developing responses to different alarm call types. Seyfarth and Cheney (1980) gathered data in the field on what elicits the alarm calls of young vervets as they grow up (Figure 1). Eagle calls given by adults are quite specific but, in contrast, infants give eagle calls to almost anything moving above in free-space, even a falling leaf, but never to a snake or a ground predator, such as a leopard. So the relationship between referents and call types sharpens with experience, as though the monkeys are developing predator-related concepts, perhaps hinting at a role for cognition in development. There are also indications of innate underpinnings to this behavior. In call production the monkeys behave as though they are innately able as youngsters, provoked to alarm calling, to divide up the world of predators into several, broad ill-defined classes leaving it to individual and social experience to bring each referent class to a focus on a particular call type as they mature. The role of innate predispositions raises some uncertainty about whether call production is a truly mindful process based on acquired internal representations of predators. On the other hand, there is a growing conviction that a great deal of human cognitive processing also has innate underpinnings (Hirschfeld & Gelman 1994; Hauser 1996; Pinker 1994). In any case, it seems probable that experience-related mentation plays a substantial role in development of how a nonhuman primate receiver responds on hearing the call (Cheney & Seyfarth 1990, 1992), even though actual call structure is minimally dependent on experience, as with all monkey and ape vocalizations. The innateness of the call morphology of monkeys is, of course, a radical contrast with speech, but the probable importance of individual experience in the emergence of call meaning, is a hint of language-like potential in monkey vocal behavior.

We have to equivocate on another aspect of the meanings of the naturally occurring vocal signals of animals. Alarm and food calls have been described as though it is reasonable to think of them as labels for things, like predators and food. In fact, we do not know what kind of label these calls represent. Our window on what they mean is provided by the responses that they elicit in others. As a result, we cannot distinguish between the labeling of an object, whether a predator or food, and a prescription for the actions relating to that object (cf. Marler 1961, 1992), a distinction that looms large in the semiotic theories of Morris (1946). One way to verbalize the message of a leopard alarm call would be "run rapidly away from bushes and up into the nearest fever tree," a good move if a leopard is around, because they hunt by stealth and ambush and cannot run or climb very rapidly. Alternatively, a more "language-like" interpretation would be that a leopard call elicits in the mind of the listener an internal representation of a leopard. Then the monkey would decide on the basis of past experience what is its best escape strategy, varying with the circumstances in which the individual finds itself. There are many important issues like this that we cannot yet address, with different implications for the kind of cognitive and brain processing that is implied. Nevertheless linkages between call and referent are more specific that we usually associate with emotional displays.

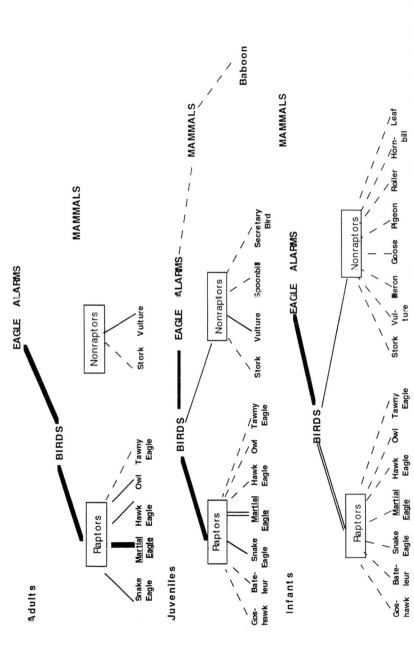

FIGURE 1. A diagrammatic summary of objects eliciting the "eagle alarm call" in adult, juvenile and infant vervet monkeys. The data were gathered in the field in Amboseli, Kenya. The width of each bar corresponds to the number of observations. At this location the martial eagle, which preys upon young vervets, is the primary referent for this call (from Seyfarth, Cheney & Marler 1980a).

Before leaving the issue of call meaning it is important to acknowledge that non-symbolic, affective signals can make a significant contribution to communication in some circumstances, as is indicated by this quotation from Norbert Wiener's 1948 book on cybernetics.

> Suppose I find myself in the woods with an intelligent savage, who cannot speak my language, and whose language I cannot speak. Even without any code of sign language common to the two of us, I can learn a great deal from him. All I need to do is to be alert to those movements when he is showing the signs of emotion or interest. I then cast my eyes around, perhaps paying attention to the direction of his glance, and fix in memory what I see or hear. It will not be long before I discover the things which seem important to him, not because he has communicated them to me by language, but because I myself have observed them (p. 157).

Thus with no other signaling elements than signs of arousal and the indexical property of gaze direction, such behavior has rich communicative potential. The theme that we are inclined to underestimate the potential of affective signaling, is echoed by Premack (1975).

> Consider two ways in which you could benefit from my knowledge of the conditions next door. I could return and tell you, 'The apples next door are ripe.' Alternatively, I could come back from next door chipper and smiling. On still another occasion I could return and tell you, 'A tiger is next door.' Alternatively, I could return mute with fright, disclosing an ashen face and quaking limbs. The same dichotomy could be arranged on numerous occasions. I could say, 'The peaches next door are ripe' or say nothing and manifest an intermediate amount of positive affect since I am only moderately fond of peaches. Likewise, I might report, 'A snake is next door,' also an intermediate amount of affect since I am less shaken by snakes than by tigers (p. 591).

Premack develops further the differences between two kinds of signaling, referential (= symbolic) and affective (= excited or aroused), suggesting that information of the first kind consists of explicit properties of the world next door while information of the second kind consists of affective states, that he assumes to be positive or negative and varying in degree. He goes on,

> Since changes in the affective states are caused by changes in the conditions next door, the two kinds of information are obviously related. In the simplest case we could arrange that exactly the condition referred to in the symbolic communication be the cause of the affective state (p. 591).

As Premack indicates, as long as there are perceptible signs of the signaler's state of arousal, and some concordance between the preferences and aversions of communicants then a significant amount of information can be transmitted by an affective system. While he explicitly restricts himself to "what" rather than "where" one may note, harking back to the Wiener quotation, that adding an indexical component to an affective signal — pointing or looking — not only indicates where, but also adds a highly specific connotation — not apple trees in general, but one in particular.

While Wiener refers to the potential of an arousal system with a single dimension, Premack implicates at least two, a dimension of positive affect concerned with attraction, and a dimension of negative affect concerned with apprehension and avoidance. While Premack seems to have had human affective signaling in mind, parallels may exist in animals. There are indications that a wide range of species, including non-human primates, tend to use high-pitched sounds in nonaggressive and fearful situations and low-pitched, harsh sounds in aggressive, and attractive situations, in accordance with what has been proscribed as a set of basic "motivational-structural rules (Morton 1977, 1982; Hauser 1993, 1996; Collias 1960), adding further to the communicative potential of affective, nonsymbolic signals. However, even with these added dimensions, emotion-based models are inadequate to explain the details of the cases of alarm calling and food calling behavior we have considered, signals satisfy the criteria for functional reference, and thus qualify as instances of symbolic communication.

Do Animals "Intend" to Communicate?

Whenever professional students of language behavior discuss the subject of linguistic reference, there is recurrent concern with the issue of intentionality. This is a philosophically complex matter that others can deal with better than I (*e.g.*, Cheney & Seyfarth 1992, 1996). I will not grapple with it here, except for one simple question. When an animal calls, does it care whether or not there is someone in range to hear the call? There are in fact some intriguing indications that presence of an "audience" can have strong effects on a signaler's behavior (Figure 2). For example, a bird that spots food, or catches sight of a predator, may or may not call, depending on whether there is a companion nearby to get the message. A male food-calling chicken will call more with an audience than without (Table 3), especially if the companion is female, and especially if she is a newcomer and thus a potential addition to his harem (Marler *et al.* 1986a, b; Evans & Marler 1994).

The modulation of a bird's calling behavior by an audience perhaps hints at an intent to communicate. Moreover, "audience effects" are not simple. They vary from one call to another, in ways that seem to be functionally adaptive, again perhaps suggesting cognitive complexities (Table 3). For example, there are strong audience effects with aerial alarm call signals that are obviously directed at companions, but none with the class of ground predator alarm calls, including mobbing calls, aimed at the predator as well as at companions (Table 3) (Marler & Evans 1996).

One possible "cognitive" interpretation of these effects of a signal audience is that animals possess an intention to communicate, and a determination to change what the other is doing. But alternative interpretations are possible. The behavior could be simply reflexive, with several reflexive circuits modulating each calling system in different ways. It would be illuminating to know whether, in cases where alarm calling behavior is audience-modulated, a calling animal is more likely to sound the alarm with an audience that is relaxed and apparently unaware of danger, and less likely to do so if it is obvious that the audience has itself already detected the danger it is in. Even then it is not clear that we could confidently infer intentionality or whether we should invoke yet another reflexive circuit. As so often happens with animal studies, it is a major and perhaps, as some believe, even an insurmountable challenge, to determine for sure what is going on in an animal's head, as indeed would be the case in ourselves, if it were not for the benefit of introspection.

Do Animals Speak in Sentences?

A primary source of the power of speech is its two-level temporal structure, what Hockett (1960) calls, the duality of patterning. The most basic requirement for speech-like behavior is a large lexicon of words that can be arranged into many differ-

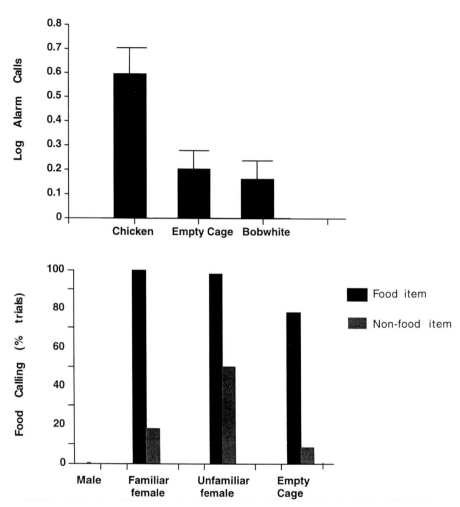

FIGURE 2. Histograms of alarm calls (left) and food calls (right) given by cockerels in response to a hawk image overhead, and to food. An adjacent cage was either empty or contained a female chicke n or a bob-white quail. Most aerial alarm calls are given with a chicken as audience. More food calls are given with a female as an audience than with a male, or with no audience. Note that deceptive food calling with a non - food item (peanut shell), occurs especially with an unfamiliar hen as an audience (after Karakashian *et al.* 1988; Marler *et al.* 1986b).

ent sentences, what Pinker (this volume) defines as a "discrete combinatorial system." It follows that there is also a need for an efficient way to produce all of these words. The most economical method is to have a small repertoire of distinct articulatory gestures or phonemes, averaging up to 40 or so in speech, with no inherent meaning in themselves, but with the potential to be sequenced in as many different ways as you choose. When meanings are attached to these sequences they become words, and when words are properly sequenced, you have a sentence, the essence of spoken language. It is useful to have different terms for these two levels of syntactical organization. The higher level, at which words and sentences are meaningful, is appropriately

TABLE 3. A chart of audience effects on the alarm and food calls of male chickens. The criteria for an effec - tive audience vary from call to call, in harmony with different functional requirements. No te there is no audience effect with the ground alarm call, which is addressed to the predator as well as to co mpanions.

	Alarm Calls		Food Calls
	Aerial alarm call	Ground alarm call	
Is there an audience effect?	Yes	No	Yes
Is audience gender relevant?	No	---	Yes
Is audience familiarity relevant?	No	---	Yes

termed "lexical syntax," involving what I call "lexicodes." The lower level, at which meaningless sounds are combined into sequences, may be termed "phonological syn- tax," involving what I call "phonocodes" for short. The distinction between "lexicod- ing" and "phonocoding" is useful in making comparisons between animal communication and language. Is there any evidence that any of these steps towards language has been taken by animals?

We can begin with lexicoding at the level of the sentence and work down in reduc- tionistic fashion. Evidence has already been presented to show that some animal sounds possess meanings in the conventional sense. However, although there are cases of animals stringing calls together, the strings all seem to mean the same thing (e g Hailman & Ficken 1987; Hailman et al 1985, 1987; Robinson 1984; Mitani & Marler 1989). There does not seem to be any recorded natural example of an animal unambiguously sequencing calls to make a sentence, where the sequence has a new meaning compiled from the meanings of its parts. Natural lexicoding appears to be a purely human phenomenon. The only animals that do anything remotely similar have been tutored by humans.

If there are no animal sentences, how about words and phonemes, or their equiva- lent? Have animals discovered the trick of phonocoding? The meaningful animal signals that I have discussed — alarm calls and food calls of monkeys and birds — all seem to come as an indivisible package. They can be repeated, and given quickly or slowly, loudly or softly, but there is no obvious analogue to phonological syntax. But if we widen the search to include animal vocalizations, not of a referential nature, but of a more classical, affective kind, impoverished in referential content, but rich in emotional content, here we can find many cases of phonological syntax. Learned birdsongs in particular provide us with an abundance of illustrations. A perusal of the literature on the structure of learned birdsongs (e.g., Kroodsma & Miller 1982), re- veals case after case where unusually large repertoires of songs are created by recom- bining in different sequences the same basic set of notes, syllables and phrases, minimal acoustic units that serve as the bird's equivalent of phonemes and syllables. Each species has its own set of phonocoding rules for creating many different songs out of these sound units. Two illustrations will serve, one simple, one more complex.

The male swamp sparrow has two or three simple two-second songs, each consist- ing of a string of identical repeated syllables. Unlike the alarm and food calls we have discussed, bird songs typically have no referential meaning. As often as not, the onset of singing is endogenously motivated, rather than being triggered by something in the environment, although certain birds, such as wood warblers, may be an exception. Songs serve as self-advertising signals, broadcasting the singer's species, sex and population membership, and the fact that he is in an emotional state of sexual and aggressive arousal. Each swamp sparrow song syllable is made up of two to six different notes, themselves meaningless, arranged in a distinctive cluster (Figure 3). The constituent notes are all drawn from a simple species-wide repertoire of six note types with a set of "phonocoding" rules for assembling them into a song (Marler & Pickert 1984). With the right combination you can describe any natural swamp sparrow song, just as you can describe the speech patterns of any language with the right combination of phonemes. Swamp sparrow song thus provides us with a clear case of phonological syntax.

The song of the winter wren is more complicated. A male has a learned repertoire of up to 5–10 song types, each up to 10 seconds in duration. Each song in a male's repertoire is different but close inspection reveals phrases that recur again and again, but in different sequences (Figure 4). Evidently when a young male learns a set of songs from adults, he breaks them down into segments, and then creates variety and enlarges the song repertoire by rearranging them in different patterns (Kroodsma 1980; Kroodsma & Momose 1991). The mistle thrush engages in very similar behavior (Marler 1959a). As in the swamp sparrow, the songs function as affective rather than symbolic signals, and the variety is generated, not to diversify meaning, but rather to maintain the interest of anyone who is listening, and to alleviate habituation.

Other songbirds take this process to extreme, creating hundreds of sequences and song types, especially, it seems, in species in which incessant male singing has assumed an important role in attracting and stimulating females. Some, such as the mockingbird and its relatives, even incorporate sounds of other species as a device for enlarging and diversifying the repertoire (Kroodsma & Miller 1982). The record is held by a male brown thrasher, with an individual song repertoire numbered in the many hundreds that he uses to bombard the female incessantly (Kroodsma & Parker 1977).

These learned birdsongs present us with one very clear parallel with speech behavior. They make extensive use of the process of syntactical recombination, but of course there is a crucial contrast with language. Generally speaking, the song sequences are not meaningfully distinct, in the referential sense. Semantically, each winter wren song means the same thing. The variety is introduced, not to enrich meaning, but to create diversity for its own sake, to alleviate boredom in singer and listener, perhaps with individual differences serving to impress the listener with the singer's virtuosity, but not to convey knowledge.

This is not, of course, to say that the great signal diversification that results is biologically insignificant. On the contrary, learned birdsongs provide an immensely rich source of cues for individual, sexual and species recognition, and for assessment of the status of the singer as a potential rival, mate, and provider of resources, as well as proffering iconic signs of a bird's current motivational state. But these are separate issues, distinct from the question of symbolic reference, which is the present concern. Also there are cases of songbirds that have functionally distinct types of singing, North American wood warblers (Lein 1972; Kroodsma 1981, 1988; Kroodsma et al. 1989; Stacier 1991; Spector 1992; Byers 1995). Often one song type is used more in conflicts between males and another is used more when males are courting females as though the two song types express different states of the singing male, one more aggressive and the other more sexual (Catchpole & Slater 1995). But I do not know of any case where different learned song types display contrasting modes of functional reference in the sense that production of one type or the other is strictly triggered by

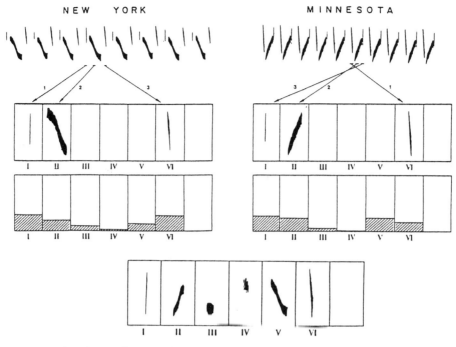

FIGURE 3. The "phonocoding" rules for male swamp sparrow song. Songs are about two seconds long, with up to 10 repeated "syllables." A syllable consists of 2–6 notes, drawn from a species-universal set of six note types. The rules for sequencing note types vary with the local dialect. Thus in the New York birds, syllables tend to begin with a type one note and end with a type six note. There is an opposite rule in Minnesota (after Marler & Pickett 1984).

encounters with a male or female. Nor is there any evidence that rearrangements of the same set of song elements have distinct referential meanings.

Learned birdsongs provide many cases of phonocoding, but none of lexicoding, an obvious and crucial contrast with language. The use of phonological syntax for generating the wonderfully diverse sound patterns of birdsong depends on the learnability of the songs. The only other corner of the animal kingdom where we find anything equivalent, apart from speech, is in the learned songs of cetaceans. Songs of the humpback whale display clear evidence of phonocoding (Payne *et al.* 1983). I know of nothing equivalent in the vast majority of animals whose vocal repertoires are innate. It is true that the pant-hooting of chimpanzees, and the songs of gibbons are made up of repeated units, but each individual has but one basic pattern. They have no song repertoires (Marler & Tenaza 1977). The only parallels I know of occur in the innate songs of some New World monkeys, which seem to indulge in phonocoding to some degree (Robinson 1979, 1984).

We can draw the inference that learned vocal behavior, evident in no primate other than humans, is an early prerequisite for the emergence of speech behavior. The probable sequence of evolutionary events thus becomes clearer. As a first step the special brain mechanisms required for vocal learning must have evolved in the immediately prehuman lineage. Then selective pressures for an enlarged vocal repertoire would have led immediately to exploitation of the potential for phonological syntax and an

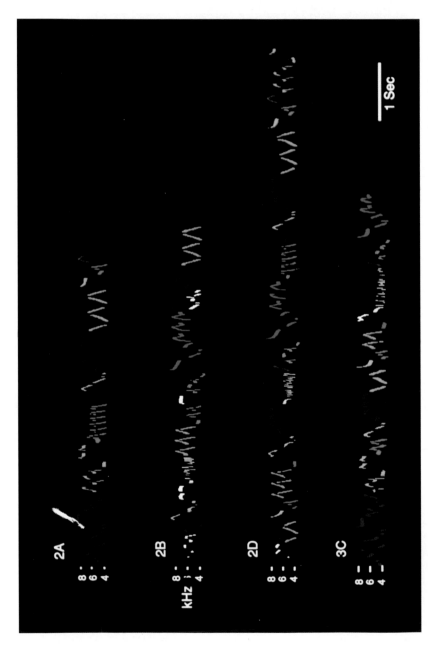

FIGURE 4. The winter wren uses phrase recombinations to create a song repertoire. Shown are three song types from the 10-song repertoire of male 2, and one song type from male 3, a neighbor, who shares phrase types with male 2 (rom Kroodsma & Momose 1991).

explosive increase in the size of the lexicon. But what gave the human brain its unique power was not just the capacity, shared with the brains of songbirds and whales, to learn and produce new sounds in an infinite number of combinations. Much more remarkable was the emergence for the first time ever of the ability to attach new meanings to newly learned sounds, and, above all, perhaps in response to the growing need for communication about tool construction and use, aided and abetted by the demands of social intelligence, the brain mechanisms necessary to retain the newly-acquired meanings as the sounds were combined into sentences, something that no other organism has ever achieved.

Conclusions

So what emerges from these reductionistically-minded speculations about the relationship between animal communication and language? We have seen that although some animal sounds do have symbolic meanings, these particular signals come as an indivisible package, with no underlying combinatorial phonocode. Phonological syntax can be found in animal signals, however, operating on basically similar principles to those underlying speech. It is largely restricted to those few animal groups — cetaceans and certain birds — in which part of the natural vocal repertoire is learned, and transmitted by cultural tradition from generation to generation. However, these naturally learned animal sounds all appear to function non-symbolically, as affective displays. So far as we know, the increased signal diversity that results in no way enriches semantic meaning, despite the great enlargement of the vocal repertoire that the capacity for phonological syntax makes possible. There is no evidence that any creature other than humans has ever taken that further step, and spoken naturally in sentences. The neuroanatomical and neurophysiological requirements for taking that further step remain an unresolved mystery. Until cognitive neuroscience provides us with some notion of the kind of circuitry that is required to learn to speak in sentences before we can understand the crucial evolutionary steps in the structure and functioning of the human brain that made language possible.

Acknowledgments

Thanks are due to Marc Hauser for thoughtful and constructive comments on the manuscript, to Donald Kroodsma for permission to use his wonderful data on winter wren song, and to three anonymous reviewers.

Literature Cited

Bastian, J. 1965. Primate signaling systems and human languages. Pages 585–606 *in* I. DeVore, ed., *Primate Behavior: Field Studies of Monkeys and Apes.* Holt, Rinehart and Winston, New York.

Benz, J.J. 1993. Food-elicited vocalizations in golden lion tamarins: Design features for representational communication. *Anim. Behav.* 45:443–455.

Benz, J.J., D.W. Leger, & J.A. French. 1992. The relation between food preference and food-elicited vocalizations in golden lion tamarins (*Leontopithecus rosalia*). *Jour. Comp. Psychol.* 106:142–149.

Boero, D.L. 1992. Alarm calling in Alpine marmot (*Marmota marmota* L.): Evidence for semantic communication. *Ethol., Ecol. Evol.* 4:125–138.

Byers, B.E. 1995. Song types. Repertoires and song variability in a population of chestnut-
sided warblers. *Condor* 97:390–401.

Catchpole, C.K. & P.J.B. Slater. 1995. *Bird Song: Biological Themes and Variations.* Cambridge University Press, Cambridge, U.K.

Cheney, D.L. & R.M. Seyfarth. 1981. Selective forces affecting the predator alarm calls of vervet monkeys. *Behaviour* 76:25–61.

————. 1985. Vervet monkey alarm calls: Manipulation through shared information? *Behaviour* 94:150–166.

————. 1988. Assessment of meaning and the detection of unreliable signals by vervet monkeys. *Anim. Behav.* 36:477–486.

————. 1990. *How Monkeys See the World: Inside the Mind of Another Species.* Chicago
University Press, Chicago.

————. 1992. Meaning, reference, and intentionality in the natural vocalizations of monkeys.
Pages 315–330 *in* T. Nishida, W.C. McGrew, P. Marler, M. Pickford, & F. de Waal, eds.,
Topics in Primatology, Vol. 1, Human Origins. Tokyo University Press, Tokyo.

Cherry, C. 1957. *On Human Communication.* John Wiley & Sons Inc., New York.

Collias, N.E. 1960. An ecological and functional classification of animal sounds. Pages
368–391 *in* W.E. Lanyon & W.N. Tavolga, eds., *Animal Sounds and Communication.*
American Institute of Biological Science Pub. No. 7, Washington, D.C.

————. 1987. The vocal repertoire of the red junglefowl: A spectrographic classification and
the code of communication. *Condor* 89:510–524.

Dittus, W. 1984. Toque macaque food calls: Semantic communication concerning food distribution in the environment. *Anim. Behav.* 32:470–477.

Elowson, A.M., P.L. Tannenbaum, & C.T. Snowdon. 1991. Food-associated calls correlate
with food preferences in cotton-top tamarins. *Anim. Behav.* 42:931–937.

Evans, C.S., L. Evans, & P. Marler. 1993. On the meaning of alarm calls: Functional reference
in an avian vocal system. *Anim. Behav.* 46:23–38.

Evans, C.S., & P. Marler. 1994. Food-calling and audience effects in male chickens, *Gallus
gallus*: Their relationships to food availability, courtship and social facilitation. *Anim. Behav.* 47:1159–1170.

————. 1995. Language and animal communication: Parallels and contrasts. Pages 341–382
in H. Roitblatt, eds., *Comparative Approaches to Cognitive Science.* MIT Press, Cambridge.

Griffin, D.R. 1992. *Animal Minds.* Chicago University Press, Chicago.

Gyger, M. & P. Marler 1988. Food calling in the domestic fowl (*Gallus gallus*): The role of external referents and deception. *Anim. Behav.* 36:358–365.

Hailman, J.P. & M.S. Ficken. 1987. Combinatorial animal communication with computable
syntax: Chick-a-dee calling qualifies as "language" by structural linguistics. *Anim. Behav.*
34:1988–1901.

Hailman, J.P., M.S. Ficken, & R.W. Ficken, 1985. The "chick-a-dee" calls of *Parus atricapil-
lus*: A recombinant system of animal communication compared with written English.
Semiotica 56:191–224.

————. 1987. Constraints on the structure of combinatorial "chick-a-dee" calls. *Ethology*
75:62–80.

Hauser, M.D. 1993. The evolution of nonhuman primate vocalizations: Effects of phylogeny,
body weight and motivational state. *Amer. Nat.* 142:528–542.

————. 1996. *The Evolution of Communication.* MIT Press, Cambridge.

Hauser, M.D. & P. Marler. 1993a. Food-associated calls to rhesus macaques (*Macaca mulatta*). I. Sociological factors. *Behav. Ecol.* 4:194–205.

——. 1993b. Food-associated calls in rhesus macaques (*Macaca mulatta*). II. Costs and benefits of call production and suppression. *Behav. Ecol.* 4:206–212.

Hauser, M.D., P. Teixidor, L. Field, & R. Flaherty, 1993. Food-elicited calls in chimpanzees: Effects of food quantity and divisibility? *Anim. Behav.* 45:817–819.

Hirschfeld, L.A. & S.A. Gelman 1994. *Mapping the Mind: Domain Specificity in Cognition and Culture.* Cambridge University Press, Cambridge, U.K.

Hockett, C.F. 1960. Logical considerations in the study of animal communication. Pages 392–430 *in* W.E. Lanyon & W.N. Tavolga, eds., *Animal Sounds and Communication.* American Institute of Biological Sciences, Washington, D.C.

Karakashian, S.J., M. Gyger, & P. Marler. 1988. Audience effects on alarm calling in chickens (*Gallus gallus*). *Jour. Comp. Psychol.* 102:129–135.

Kroodsma, D.E. 1980. Winter Wren singing behavior: A pinnacle of song complexity. *Condor* 82:357–365.

——. 1981. Geographical variation and functions of song types in warblers (Parulidae). *Auk* 98:743–751.

——. 1988. Song types and their use: developmental flexibility of the male Blue-winged Warbler. *Ethology* 79:235–247.

Kroodsma, D.E., R.C. Bereson, B.E. Byers, & E. Minear. 1989. Use of song types by the Chestnut-sided Warbler: Evidence for both intra- and inter-sexual functions. *Canad. Jour. Zool.* 67:447–456.

Kroodsma, D.E. & E.H. Miller, 1982. *Acoustic Communication in Birds.* Academic Press, New York.

Kroodsma, D.E. & H. Momose 1991. Songs of the Japanese population of the Winter Wren (*Troglodytes troglodytes*). *Condor* 93:424–432.

Kroodsma, D.E. & L.D. Parker. 1977. Vocal virtuosity in the Brown Thrasher. *Auk* 94:783–785.

Lancaster, J. 1965. *Primate Behavior and the Emergence of Human Culture.* Holt, Rinchart Winston, New York.

Luria, A. 1982. *Language and Cognition.* MIT Press, Cambridge.

Macedonia, J.M. 1991. What is communicated in the antipredator calls of lemurs? Evidence from playback experiments with ring-tailed and ruffed lemurs. *Ethology* 86:177–190.

Marin, O., Schwarz, M.F. & E.M. Saffran. 1979. Origins and distribution of language. Pages 179–213 *in* M.S. Gazzaniga, ed., *Handbook of Behavioral Biology II.* Plenum Press, New York.

Marler, P. 1955. Characteristics of some animal calls. *Nature* 176:6–7.

——. 1959a. Developments in the study of animal communication. Pages 150–206 and 329-335 *in* P.R. Bell, ed., *Darwin's Biological Work.* Cambridge University Press, Cambridge, U.K.

——. 1959b. The voice of the chaffinch and its function as a language. *Ibis* 98:231–261.

——. 1961. The logical analysis of animal communication. *Jour. Theoret. Biol.* 1:295–317.

——. 1992. Functions of arousal and emotion in primate communication: A semiotic approach. Pages 235–248 *in* T. Nishida, W.C. McGrew, P. Marler, M. Pickford, & F.B.M. de-Waal, eds., *Topics in Primatology, Vol 1, Human Origins.* University of Tokyo Press, Tokyo.

Marler, P. & C.S. Evans. 1997. Animal sounds and human faces: Do they have anything in common? Pages 133–157 *in* J.A. Russell & J.M. Fernandez-Dols, eds., *The Psychology of Facial Expression.* Cambridge University Press, Cambridge, U.K.

Marler, P., A. Dufty, & R. Pickert. 1986a. Vocal communication in the domestic chicken: I. Does a sender communicate information about the quality of a food referent to a receiver? *Anim. Behav.* 34:188–193.

———. 1986b. Vocal communication in the domestic chicken: II. Is a sender sensitive to the presence and nature of a receiver? *Anim. Behav.* 34:194–198.

Marler, P., C.S. Evans, & M.D. Hauser. 1992. Animal signals? Reference, motivation or both? Pages 66–86 *in* H. Papoucek, U. Jurgens, & M. Papoucek, eds., *Nonverbal Vocal Communication: Comparative and Developmental Approaches*. Cambridge University Press, Cambridge, U.K.

Marler, P. & C.S. Evans. 1996. Bird calls: Just emotional displays or something more? *Ibis* 138:26–331.

Marler, P. & R. Pickert. 1984. Species-universal microstructure in the learned song of the swamp sparrow (*Melospiza georgiana*). *Anim. Behav.* 32:673–689.

Marler P. & R. Tenaza. 1977. Signaling behavior of apes, with special reference to vocalization. Pages 965–1033 *in* T. Sebeok, ed., *How Animals Communicate*. Indiana University Press, Bloomington.

Mitani, J.C. & P. Marler. 1989. A phonological analysis of male gibbon singing behavior. *Behaviour* 109:20–45.

Morris, C. 1946. *Signs, Language and Behavior*. Prentice Hall, New York.

Morton, E.S. 1977. On the occurrence and significance of motivation-structural rules in some birds and mammal sounds. *Amer. Nat.* 111:855–869.

———. 1982. Grading, discreteness, redundancy, and motivational-structural rules. Pages 183–212 *in* D. Kroodsma & E.H. Miller, eds., *Acoustic Communication in Birds*, Vol. 1. Academic Press, New York.

Myers, R.E. 1976. Comparative neurology of vocalization and speech: Proof of a dichotomy. Pages 745–757 *in* S.R. Harnad, H.D. Steklis, & L. Lancaster, eds., *Origins and Evolution of Language and Speech*. New York Academy of Sciences, New York.

Payne, K., P. Tyack, & R. Payne. 1983. Progressive changes in the songs of humpback whales (Megaptera novaeangliae): A detailed analysis of two seasons in Hawaii. Pages 9–57 *in* R. Payne, ed., *Communication and Behavior of Whales*. AAAS Selected Symposia Series. Westview Press, Boulder.

Pinker, S. 1994. *The Language Instinct*. William Morrow and Company Inc., New York.

Premack, D. 1975. On the origins of language. Pages 591–605 *in* M.S. Gazzaniga & C.B. Blakemore, eds., Handbook of Psychobiology. Academic Press, New York.

Robinson, J.G. 1979. An analysis of the organization of vocal communication in the titi monkey *Callicebus moloch*. *Zeits. Tierpsychol.* 49:381–405.

———. 1984. Syntactic structures in the vocalizations of wedge-capped capuchin monkeys. *Cebus nigrivittatus*. *Behaviour* 90:46–79.

Rowell, T.E. & Hinde, R.A. 1962. Vocal communication in rhesus monkey (*Macaca mulatta*). *Proc. Zool. Soc. Lond.* 138:279–294.

Sebeok, T.A. 1976. *Contributions to the Doctrine of Signs*. Indiana University, Bloomington.

Seyfarth, R.M. & D.L. Cheney. 1980. The ontogeny of vervet monkey alarm-calling behavior: A preliminary report. *Zeits. Tierpsychol.* 54:37–56.

Seyfarth, R.M., D.L. Cheney, & P. Marler. 1980a. Monkey responses to three different alarm calls: Evidence of predator classification and semantic communication. *Science* 210:801–803.

Seyfarth, R.M., D.L. Cheney, & P. Marler. 1980b. Vervet monkey alarm calls: Semantic communication in a free-ranging primate. *Anim. Behav.* 28:1070–1094.

Smith, W.J. 1981. Referents of animal communication. *Anim. Behav.* 29:1273–1275.

Spector, D.A. 1992. Wood-warbler song systems: A review of paruline singing behaviors. *Curr. Orinthol.* 9:199–238.

Stacier, C.A. 1989. Characteristics, use and significance of two singing behaviors in Grace's warbler (*Dendroica graciae*). *Auk* 106:49–63.

Struhsaker, T.T. 1967. Auditory communication among vervet monkeys (*Cercopithecus aethiops*). Pages 281–324 *in* S.A. Altmann, ed., *Social Communication Among Primates.* Chicago University Press, Chicago.

Tamura, N. & H.-S. Young. 1993. Vocalizations in response to predators in three species of Malaysian *Callosciurus* (Sciuridae). *Jour. Mammal.* 74:703–714.

Walters, J.R. 1990. Anti-predator behavior of lapwings: Field evidence of discriminative abilities. *Wilson Bull.* 102:49–70.

Wiener, N. 1948. *Cybernetics.* Wiley and Sons, New York.

Zivin, G., ed. 1985. *The Development of Expressive Behavior.* Academic Press, New York.

Zuberbuhler, K., R. Noe, & R.M. Seyfarth. 1997. Diana monkey long-distance calls: Messages for conspecifics and predators. *Anim. Behav.* 53:589–604.

The Foundations of Human Language

Leslie C. Aiello
Department of Anthropology
University College London
Gower Street
London WC1E 6BT, UK

The foundations of modern human language are often sought in the communication capabilities of our closest living relatives, the chimpanzees. Many lines of modern research suggest, however, that fully developed human language did not appear until after about 500,000 years ago, while at least 5 million years separates us from the last common ancestor we share with the chimpanzees. It would be naive to think that modern human language developed directly from a chimpanzee type of communication system without significant intermediary stages.

It is argued that the most important intermediary stage in the development of modern human language had little to do initially with vocal communication. Rather it was related to a major transition in early human lifestyle that took place about two million years ago in Africa. At this time our ancestors moved from a forested, or woodland, environment where they were partially tree-living to a more open-country lifestyle. This new environment required new biological and behavioral adaptations, many of which are directly related to vocal communication. These included living in larger groups, having larger home ranges, and adopting a different diet and locomotor pattern. During this period there was also a major increase in brain size. When these adaptations are viewed in the context of the archaeological and paleontological records and of other fields such as developmental psychology and neuroanatomy, a picture emerges of a human ancestor with preadaptations what would better suit it to the later development of modern language than any living primate.

In the search for the foundations of modern human language, one must clearly distinguish between human speech and human language. Human speech is defined as the sounds that are characteristic of human language. The ability to produce human speech is dependent on the unique structure of the human vocal tract (Figure 1, see also Aiello & Dean 1990). Humans have a muscular tongue, a distinctively shaped jaw and a larynx which is located low in the throat (Lieberman & Crelin 1971; Lieberman *et al.* 1992; Duchin 1990). Humans also have the neurological coordination that permits the necessary complex articulatory movements of the jaw, lips and tongue in respect to the teeth, palate and pharynx. This allows us to produce the wide range of

The Origin and Diversification of Language
Editors, N.G. Jablonski & L.C. Aiello

Memoirs of the California Academy of Sciences
Number 24, Copyright ©1998

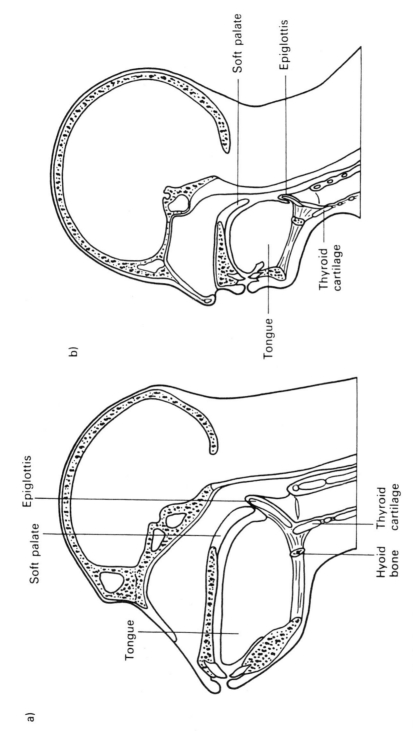

FIGURE 1. Midsagittal section through the heads of (a) a chimpanzee and (b) a modern human. The position of the thyroid cartilage indicates the position of the larynx in the neck. Note that in the human the soft palate does not contact the epiglottis. This is an important feature in the production of human speech because the tongue forms the anterior wall of the ascending pharynx (throat). It can change the shape of the throat to produce different vowel sounds. Reprinted with permission from Aiello & Dean (1990).

vowels and consonants characteristic of human speech. The production of human speech is also not innate. It requires voluntary learning to control and to coordinate the vocal apparatus.

In contrast to speech, human language is our ability to communicate vocally. It is characterized by three distinctive features. Firstly, human language uses a finite number of sounds to generate an infinite number of meanings (Deacon 1992). Sounds, or phonemes, are combined into words and words are combined into sentences. The order of the sound, or syntax, is fundamentally important. Second, human language is symbolic in nature. The individual phonemes, words or sentences are arbitrary in relation to the meaning that is being conveyed. And third, the sounds are not tied to immediate events. This involves off-line thinking where real or imaginary events can be discussed with reference to both the past and the future (Bickerton 1990, 1995).

In this paper, I will argue that these two aspects of human vocal communication, the ability to produce human speech and the ability to produce human language, did not appear in our evolutionary history at the same time or for the same reasons. Many of the unique anatomical features involved in the ability to produce human speech, as well as some of the cognitive precursors of human language, significantly preceded the appearance of fully developed modern human language involving syntax, symbolic reference and off-line thinking. Modern human language is built on foundations that extend back over two million years into our evolutionary history. As we will find, many of these foundations are the result of adaptations that initially had little, if anything, to do with vocal communication.

The Search for the Foundations of Language

In the search for the foundations of human language, a logical place to begin is with the first definite evidence for its appearance. Many authors have argued that the only direct evidence for symbolic human language is the presence in the archaeological record of evidence for symbolic thinking. The focus has been on apparent differences between the material remains left by the Neanderthals and anatomically modern humans in Europe (White 1982; Chase & Dibble 1987; Mellars 1991; Noble & Davidson 1991; Davidson & Noble 1993; Milo & Quiatt 1993). In this volume Mellars provides a particularly clear discussion of the virtual lack of convincing evidence for explicit symbolic thinking in Neanderthals. He also notes that the Neanderthals apparently lacked any interest in the visual appearance of the tools they made. Different types of tools, which were apparently used for different purposes, grade into one another without clear-cut divisions. Mellars suggests that this might indicate that Neanderthals lacked a highly structured vocabulary which would provide names for distinct artifact types. The absence of complexity in many other aspects of Neanderthal culture also suggests to him that Neanderthals may have been deficient in the capacity to organize and structure their activities. The greater degree of both chronological and spatial variation in technology associated with anatomically modern humans, in contrast to the Neanderthals, suggests to him that early modern humans had more sharply defined ethnic divisions. These last two points are significant because language is used to transmit rules of complex behavior and specifically defined cultural traditions.

The apparent difference between Neanderthal and anatomically modern human archaeological remains and inferred linguistic and cognitive abilities are particularly relevant in the context of newly published genetic evidence. Krings and his coworkers (Krings *et al.* 1997) suggest that all living modern humans are more closely related to each other than any of us are to the Neanderthals. Their evidence also suggests that the split leading to the Neanderthals on the one hand and to modern humans on the other occurred about 600,000 years ago. The line leading to modern humans, therefore, would have been separate from the line leading to Neanderthals for a significant length of time. Different cognitive processes, possibly including language, could have developed in the two lineages. This possibility is interesting in the context of new analyses of Neanderthal brain size. Whereas previous work emphasized the unusually large brain sizes of the Neanderthals, new estimates of their body masses tell a slightly different story (Ruff *et al.* 1997). The large Neanderthal brains are smaller than those of modern humans in relation to their considerable body masses.

It is possible that the Neanderthals may not have had a system of vocal communication characterized by any or all of the factors that define modern human language. This is particularly interesting because Neanderthals did apparently have a vocal apparatus that would have been compatible with the production of the full range of sounds necessary for human speech. The best evidence for this is the existence of a Neanderthal hyoid bone from the site of Kebara in Israel (Arensburg *et al.* 1989, 1990). This hyoid is fundamentally modern in form. It implies that the Neanderthal larynx was located low in the throat, in a position that would be consistent with the production of the full range of sounds characteristic of human speech (Figure 1).

Analysis of the Neanderthal jaw also shows that it was shaped in such a way as to give the muscles that move the tongue proper leverage. Duchin (1990) has argued that unless the jaw is short and broad the tongue simply cannot be positioned in the oral cavity in the variety of ways necessary to produce the full range of sounds characteristic of human speech. In her analyses Neanderthal jaws fall clearly within the human range of variation. Assuming that Neanderthals had the necessary cortical control of their tongues, there is no anatomical reason why they could not have produced human speech. Because of the unusually large Neanderthal nasal passages however, their speech would most probably have had a considerable nasal quality.

This evidence for Neanderthal speech, and particularly for the inferred low position of the Neanderthal larynx, directly contradicts the work of Lieberman and his colleagues (see particularly Lieberman *et al.* 1992; Lieberman & Crelin 1971). For more than twenty years they have argued that the Neanderthals were different from modern humans and similar to all other primates in having a very high larynx and a vocal tract incapable of producing the full range of human speech. Not only does the previously cited evidence argue against this interpretation, but also the conclusions of Lieberman and his coworkers have been repeatedly criticized on the basis of a variety of other anatomical criteria (see particularly Schepartz 1993; Houghton 1993; McCarthy & D. Lieberman, 1997; but see P. Lieberman *et al.*1992, 1994).

The evidence presented here is consistent with other arguments that have been made for the appearance of the modern human vocal tract even earlier in our evolutionary history. The descent of the larynx and the change of the shape of the jaw, as well as other necessary anatomical and behavioral foundations for human language, may have been simple consequences of fundamental morphological and lifestyle changes that accompanied the evolution of *Homo ergaster* (early African *Homo erectus*) almost two million years ago (Aiello 1996a, 1996b).

Anatomical Foundations For Human Speech
in the Plio-Pleistocene

Homo ergaster appears in the fossil record at about 1.8 million years ago and was the first known hominin to have resembled modern humans in its overall body proportions, and particularly in the length of its legs in relation to its inferred body mass (Walker & Leakey 1993). It is also the first known hominin to be a dedicated biped, lacking all of the features in its postcranial skeleton that indicated arboreal locomotion in the earlier australopithecines.

Homo ergaster occupied substantially different habitats than those occupied by earlier hominins (Cachel & Harris 1995; Reid 1997). In particular, *Homo ergaster* lived in drier, more open (savanna) parts of the environment (Reid 1997; Stanley 1992). Earlier australopithecine species are found in fairly wooded, well-watered regions, while *Paranthropus* (*P. aethiopicus, P. robustus, P. boisei*), who first appeared about 2.6 million years ago and survived until about 1.4 million years ago, occupied both wooded and open environments, but always near wetlands (Reid 1997).

Homo ergaster was also the first hominin to have relatively small teeth (McHenry 1988) and jaws (Wood & Aiello, in press), reflecting a fundamental change in diet. This new diet most probably involved significantly greater amounts of animal-based products. Such a change in diet is a necessary consequence of the increase in brain size observed in early *Homo* (Aiello & Wheeler 1995; Aiello 1997; Aiello in press). The brain is very expensive in metabolic terms, requiring per unit mass over 22 times the amount of energy required by an equivalent amount of muscle tissue. In order to grow and maintain a large brain, its energy requirements have to be met. Humans do not have an unusually high basal metabolic rate to provide energy for our large brains. Rather we have enough energy for our relatively large brains because one of our other energetically expensive organs, the gut, is relatively small. (Aiello & Wheeler 1995; Aiello 1997). A reduction in gut size relative to body size is only possible by moving to higher-quality and more easy to digest food. In the case of our early ancestors, high quality food that would have been readily available would have been animal-based products such as meat, fat and bone marrow. At this stage in human evolution there is no evidence of any type of food preparation, such as cooking, that would enhance the digestibility of more difficult to digest foods.

Direct archaeological evidence for a major shift in diet comes from a number of different sources. The microwear on the stone tools indicates that they were used at least in part for the acquisition and preparation of meat, fat and marrow (Keeley & Toth 1981; Bunn 1981; Potts & Shipman 1981). Analysis of the animal bones left in the archaeological sites also shows that the hominins were better able to control parts of the landscape and to protect carcasses from scavengers (Monahan 1996). A greater variety of game animals are represented in the sites and the animal bone is more fragmentary (Isaac 1975; Cachel & Harris 1995). Cachel and Harris (1995) note that the large body size in *Homo ergaster,* which is 50% greater than the average body mass of the australopithecines, also may reflect increasing dietary protein from animal-based sources.

These major morphological and lifestyle changes characteristic of *Homo ergaster* are fundamental to both human speech and human language. The change in shape and robusticity of the jaw resulting from dietary change is particularly important (Aiello 1996a, 1996b). In Duchin's (1990) analysis of jaw shape in relation to speech production, she concluded that Middle Pleistocene *Homo erectus*, as well as the Neanderthals, could have produced human speech. More recently, Oniko (n.d.) has demonstrated that other early members of the genus *Homo* would also have had the necessary jaw proportions. In contrast, none of the australopithecines or paranthropines would have had jaw proportions compatible with the production of the full range of human speech sounds.

The small jaw and less projecting face of *Homo ergaster* may also be associated directly with the descent of the larynx from its high ape-like position to a position lower in the throat. In bipedal hominins, the head is balanced on the vertebral column which lies under the skull in a more anterior position than it occupies in the apes. In *Homo ergaster* the anterior position of the vertebral column (and foramen magnum) together with the reduction of the face and jaws may simply have squeezed the larynx into its lower position in the throat (Aiello 1996a, 1996b). Alternatively, reduction in the size of the face and the jaw may actually require the descent of the larynx.

Acoustic features of animal calls communicate cues of individual- and kinship-related identity (Owren 1996). These identity features do not involve complex articulations of the vocal apparatus, but rather result from minor individual variations in the actual vocal tract anatomy that produce variations in resonance. A short face reduces the length of the vocal tract. The shorter the vocal tract, the higher and more widely spaced are the resonance frequencies, and the less effective are the resonance frequencies in providing cues to individual identity (Owren 1996). A lower larynx may simply result from the need to maintain a minimum overall vocal tract length to preserve the identity-signaling system (Owren 1996). This, together with the advantageous shape of the jaw resulting from dietary change, would have provided one of the first building blocks in the anatomical foundations for the evolution of human speech Neither of these features would have been selected for in the context of human speech but would have been consequences of the dietary changes that were taking place at this time in human evolution.

By the Early Pleistocene *Homo ergaster* would, therefore, have had at least two anatomical prerequisites for human speech, a low larynx and an advantageously shaped jaw. But what was the linguistic ability of *Homo ergaster*? If these hominins did have the morphological adaptations outlined above, were they communicating vocally in any way that modern humans might recognize as language? If not, when did fully developed modern human language appear and what factors underlie this remarkable form of vocal communication?

Tool Making and the Cognitive Foundations
for Human Language

One of the problems in reconstructing the linguistic capabilities of our early ancestors is that we have no living analogue. *Homo ergaster* was unlike living apes in anatomy and habitat preference. Likewise these hominins were unlike modern humans.

One of the fundamental differences between living apes and modern humans is that apes live in the present time. They are unreflective, concrete in their actions and situation bound. Their cognitive capabilities are episodic in nature (Donald 1991). Any linguistic abilities that they might acquire through laboratory teaching by humans, are immediate, short-term responses to the environment. This contrasts with human abstract symbolic memory. Our consciousness allows us to think about and act on events in the past and plan for the future. It also allows us to engage in collective plans and representations with others.

One of the first steps in the evolution of language is to break the episodic nature of cognition and to acquire the ability to produce conscious, self-initiated, representational acts. The first tangible evidence of this cognitive breakthrough may well be the Acheulian tool tradition (Wynn 1991; Donald 1991). The Acheulian tool tradition first appears in Africa at about 1.4 million years ago (Asfaw *et al.* 1992). It persists with an impressive degree of stylistic uniformity in Africa and the western half of Eurasia until about 150,000 years ago when it is replaced by more elaborate Middle Paleolithic stone tool industries (Gowlett 1992). It is characterized by well formed, symmetrical handaxes that have been interpreted to reflect the technical demands of a diet based on a higher proportion of animal-based foodstuffs (Shipman & Walker 1989). In a sense, the Acheulian would have provided the artificial claws and teeth allowing the early hominins to butcher the animals that they either hunted or scavenged.

The Acheulian represents a level of cognitive ability over and above the earlier Olduwan tool tradition (Wynn 1991). Acheulian hand axes could not have been produced by trial and error as could Olduwan chopping tools. Rather they would require a clear conscious idea of the shape of the tool and the sequence of tool-making action to achieve that shape. This would have involved a level of intentionality and autocueing that is not apparent in the production of the earlier Olduwan tools and is unknown in modern primates. The distribution and character of the slightly earlier stone tools from the Okote Member of the Koobi Fora Formation, Kenya (*ca.* 1.6 million years ago) also show evidence of anticipation of a future need for stone and flexible manufacturing strategies based on the size of the raw material available (Rogers 1997).

In Donald's (1991, 1993) view the cognitive ability reflected in the Acheulian is part of a larger complex which he terms mimetic culture. He sees mimesis as a revolution in motor skill that "rests on the ability to produce conscious, self-initiated, representational acts that are intentional but not linguistic" (Donald 1991:168). The main element in mimesis is the ability to intentionally re-represent a situation and reflect on it. This can be done individually, such as rehearsing an event to one's self as in the manufacture of an Acheulian tool. Importantly, it also can be done in the context of social communication.

Group Size, Social Intelligence and the Cognitive Foundations of Human Language

In nonhuman primates vocalization is primarily controlled by the limbic system and the cingulate gyrus. One of the first steps in the evolution of human language would be to give voluntary control to the modulation of vocalizations that are already so important in primate sociality (Orwen 1996). The ability to regulate the volume, pitch, and tone of the voice for emphasis would have been an important initial step in the ability to produce the rapid, consciously controlled, vocalizations necessary for human language (Donald 1991).

Possible selection pressures for increased vocal mimesis may lie with the unique open habitat and dietary transition characteristic of *Homo ergaster*. Those nonhuman primates that today live in open environments tend to have larger group sizes than those living in forested environments (Foley 1987). Reasons for this might include the increased predator pressure in such open environments or the competition with mammalian carnivores for meat (Cachel & Harris 1995). Protection from both of these dangers would be gained through larger group sizes (Aiello & Dunbar 1993). Large group sizes, however, pose problems of social cohesion and intragroup competition. Nonhuman primates reinforce their social networks through mutual grooming and there is a strong correlation between group size and time spent in grooming behavior. Primates cannot spend more than about 20% of their daily time budgets in grooming and still have time for other necessary activities such as feeding, resting or traveling (Dunbar 1992, 1993, 1994). As group sizes increase and more grooming time is required, other activities suffer and this ultimately affects individual survival and fitness. Because some primate calls already have the strong social function of signaling individual identity (Orwen 1996), the conscious exaggeration of calls for more emphasis in the context of vocal grooming (Aiello & Dunbar 1993) is a logical first step in vocal mimesis (Donald 1991). Furthermore, larger group sizes have costs in terms of intragroup competition for resources. Brain size (neocortex ratio), group size and use of deception all intercorrelate strongly in higher primates (Byrne & Whitten 1992; Byrne 1996). Vocal mimesis may have evolved to allow the unemotional use of calls to manipulate the behavior of others.

One other aspect of *Homo ergaster* morphology which may be important in the context of an early generalized mimetic adaptation is the locomotor pattern of these hominins. Dedicated bipedal locomotion with a total absence of any specific adaptations for tree living, is first apparent in *Homo ergaster*. This type of locomotion would have freed not only the hands but also the entire upper body from locomotor function. Furthermore, the change in body proportions and reduction of the gut would have provided these early hominins with a waist and rendered the upper body much more mobile than is inferred for the earlier australopithecines (Schmid 1991; Aiello & Wheeler 1995). The motor-vocal cross modalities that are postulated for mimesis at this stage in human evolution with re-representation and autocueing, which would essentially be replaying events in the mind, may well have also heralded the first appearance of rhythm and use of the entire body to reenact, or rehearse, events (Donald 1991, 1993). In the first instance this may simply have taken the form of rehearsing the movements used in stone tool making or playing with vocalizations in the context of vocal mimesis. It could have rapidly come to involve the use of the whole body. The ubiquitous occurrence of rhythm, dance and song in all human cultures today may attest to the deep evolutionary roots of this uniquely human ability in the dietary and habitat transition of our early *Homo ergaster* ancestors. The cross modal mimetic ability may also underlie the later evolving human ability to communicate symbolically using a variety of modalities (voice, gesture and also the written word).

Primate Social Intelligence and the Evolution of Language

An important question is why other primates living in large group sizes in open habitats have not also developed vocal mimesis? The answer may simply be that they did not also undergo a major shift in their diet of the type postulated for *Homo ergaster*. They would have not undergone the anatomical changes connected with adoption of a higher quality diet nor would they have been subjected to the complexities of social organization presupposed by this dietary transition. These social complexities are not simply the elaborate mental maps or more sophisticated organization necessary for successful hunting and scavenging postulated by those who normally argue a connection between feeding behavior and cognitive evolution (Parker & Gibson 1979; Clutton-Brock & Harvey 1980; Gibson 1986). There are fundamental changes in interpersonal relationships connected with the dietary transition (Hawkes *et al.* 1997, 1997a, 1997b; Aiello in press). These fundamental changes are required by the basic fact that a high quality diet composed at least in part of animal-based products would not be directly accessible to weanlings (Hawkes *et al.* 1997, 1997a, 1997b).

In nonhuman primates, weanlings and juveniles tend to forage for themselves. Both they and their mothers are limited to resources which can be managed without undue skill or learning. A high quality diet which included significant amounts of meat, fat or marrow, or for that matter plant food requiring extensive extraction or preparation, would presuppose regular provisioning of the weanling. This implies a significant amount of mother-infant food sharing as well as increased maternal investment to train the infant to efficiently obtain the food resource. The period of maternal investment in the offspring would be extended significantly past the weaning period resulting in increased energetic stress on the female as she came into her next fertile period. This has at least two important implications for human evolution.

The first implication is that it opens up the opportunity for kin other than the mother (particularly grandmothers) to enhance their own reproductive fitness by provisioning the weanling. Hawkes and her coworkers argue that this may well be the driving factor behind the evolution of the complex of unique human life-history features including the menopause and extended longevity as well as a relatively late age at maturity and the relatively high level of human fertility in relation to the apes (Hawkes *et al.* 1997b; submitted).

The second important implication revolves around the fact that there was undoubtedly a higher level of adult mortality in human prehistory than in the present day. Many (most) females would not have had surviving senior female kin to aid in provisioning. Under these circumstances, hominin mothers would have had a strong incentive to encourage provisioning from other members of the group and particularly from males (Aiello in press; Key & Aiello in press). Aspects of female reproductive physiology such as concealed ovulation, continuous sexual receptivity and reproductive seasonality would be expected to lead to improved levels of attentiveness and investment by the males in the females (Dunbar 1988; Ridley 1989; Power *et al.* 1997). This would also be expected to increase the levels of deceptive behavior between the sexes. This is because males and females have fundamentally different and potentially conflicting reproductive strategies (Trivers 1972). Whereas females are limited in the number of children they can conceive, bear and raise to maturity, males are only limited by the number of females that they can inseminate. There would be a strong incentive for females to use deceptive tactics to encourage provisioning from the male (in possible return for sexual access) while at the same time there would be an equally strong incentive for the males to use deceptive behavior to gain sexual access to the female without engaging in the levels of provisioning that might be to her best benefit. A transition to a high quality diet would therefore be expected to increase the level of interpersonal interaction between members of the group and at the same time provide a strong selective pressure for enhanced levels of social intelligence above the level observed in living nonhuman primates.

Social intelligence is a fundamental prerequisite for the origin of fully developed modern human language. There are similarities in reasoning processes or procedures between primate social intelligence and the computational basis of language processing including both the semantic aspects of language and syntax (Worden in press). Social intelligence has all the fundamental features of language meanings. It is structured, complex and open-ended, discrete valued, extended in space and time, and dependent on sensory data of all modalities.

In Worden's view, primates store social events as scripts (or procedures). The learning of general rules about events results from the comparison of these scripts. The level of social intelligence characterizing a particular species is determined by the complexity of the scripts or procedures that can be stored in the brain. This complexity is determined by both the size of the brain and its design features. For example, the procedures that allow primates with basic social intelligence (such as the vervet monkeys) to recognize other individuals would also enable them to recognize and assign meaning to alarm calls. The more complex social intelligence of the chimpanzees, involving the controversial presence of Theory of Mind (the ability to understand what another individual is thinking) (Povinelli & Preuss 1995), provides the procedural basis for the linguistic capabilities evident in laboratory trained animals. The highly developed social intelligence of humans, involving higher order Theory of Mind, provides the procedural basis for syntax. The procedures that primates use for complex social planning and anticipation are, therefore, one and the same as those operations that provide the cognitive foundations for human language learning and understanding.

Linguistic Capabilities of *Homo ergaster* and Beyond

The transition to a higher quality diet would have had fundamental morphological and cognitive implications for the later development of modern human language. The morphological adaptations are driven by the reduction of the face and jaw that correlates with the reduced chewing requirements of a higher quality animal-based diet. Not only can this be directly related to the lowering of the larynx and the potential ability to articulate a wider range of vowel sounds, but it can also be related to a greater potential for facial expression (Lieberman 1984). The different geometry of the *Homo ergaster* lower face would be expected to have altered the insertion points of the facial muscles resulting in a greater range of facial expression. At the same time, the tools required by the new diet imply a level of cognitive ability that exceeds that seen in living apes or inferred for the earlier australopithecines. As reflected in the Acheulian tool tradition, this cognitive ability would have begun to break the episodic nature of culture and allow our evolutionary ancestors to re-represent and reflect on past events. If Donald is correct in the cross-modal nature of mimesis, we would also expect at this time to have the beginnings of conscious control of vocalizations. Initially this would have only involved the ability to modulate and extend existing vocalizations for purposes of social control or manipulation.

On the basis of this reasoning the linguistic capability of *Homo ergaster* may have included more structure than is apparent in the symbolic communication of laboratory trained chimpanzees. This conclusion is based on the inferred more complex level of social intelligence required as a consequence of the dietary-based fundamental changes in social organization. It is also fair to assume that there would have been a wider range of vocalizations available to the early hominins and that these would have been under more cortical control than in modern nonhuman primates. There is no clear evidence as to the nature of the symbolic content of these vocalizations. Evidence from laboratory trained chimpanzees suggests that they have the capability of learning a respectable lexicon and it would be reasonable to assume that the early hominins would have had at least this ability.

The best evidence we have for the evolution of fully developed modern human language from this basis is the rapid increase of brain size that gets underway about

500,000 years ago, over one million years after the first appearance of *Homo ergaster* (Deacon 1992; Aiello 1996b; Ruff *et al.* 1997). The enlarging human brain would not only provide increased memory capacity for an expanded lexicon but also for the required procedural templates underlying social intelligence and syntactically based language. The prefrontal cortex of the brain, which is particularly large in humans as a result of overall brain expansion (Semendeferi *et al.* 1997), is specifically responsible for many features of language production and comprehension as well as the unique human ability to reflect on our own mental states and those of others (Theory of Mind) (Povinelli & Preuss 1995).

At present there is no clear reason for this runaway evolution of brain size with its implications for language evolution and social intelligence. There is also no clear idea of how the Neanderthals fit into this picture. Aiello and Dunbar (1993) have speculated that the expansion of the brain may well have to do with increased group size and intergroup competition, a view which is shared by many others in the field (*e.g.*, Donald 1991; Pinker 1994). However, one certain thing is that the evolution of increased social intelligence would be closely linked with the evolution of language. The reason for this is simply that an increased ability to communicate symbolically would be tied with the increased ability to cheat. Higher level social intelligence (Theory of Mind) is without a doubt an ability to read and manipulate others in order to protect one's self against manipulators. The procedural templates involved in this increased social intelligence would be the same procedural templates involved in the ability to generate more complex linguistic structures. The one would go hand-in-hand with the other and both abilities would be expected to evolve rapidly in evolutionary time.

Acknowledgments

I would like to thank the Paul L. and Phyllis Wattis Foundation Endowment and the California Academy of Sciences for making the 1997 Wattis Symposium on *The Origin and Diversification of Language* possible. I would also like to thank Dr. Nina Jablonski for inviting me to participate in this symposium. I would also like to thank the following people for discussion and criticism of the arguments presented here: Robin Dunbar, Kathleen Gibson, Catherine Key, Bob Martin, Paul Mellars, James O'Connell, Michael Orwen, Camilla Power, Todd Preuss, Peter Wheeler, Elizabeth Whitcomb, and Robert Worden.

Literature Cited

Aiello, L.C. 1996a. Hominine preadaptations for language and cognition. Pages 269–288 *in* P. Mellars & K. Gibson, eds., *Modelling the early human mind*, McDonald Institute Monograph Series, Cambridge, U.K.

————. 1996b. Terrestriality, bipedalism and the origin of language. Pages 269–289 *in* W.G. Runciman, J. Maynard Smith & R.I.M. Dunbar, eds., *Evolution of social behaviour patterns in primates and man,* (Proceedings of the British Academy, vol. 88), The British Academy, London, U.K.

————. 1997. Brains and guts in human evolution: the expensive tissue hypothesis. *Brazil. Jour. Genet.* 20:141-148

————. in press. The expensive tissue hypothesis and the evolution of the human adaptive niche: A study in comparative anatomy *in* J. Bayley, ed., *Proceedings of the Science in Ar-*

chaeology Conference. HBMC Archaeology Reports Series, English Heritage, London, U.K.

Aiello, L.C. & C. Dean. 1990. *An Introduction to Human Evolutionary Anatomy*. Academic Press, London, U.K.

Aiello, L.C. & R.I.M. Dunbar. 1993. Neocortex size, group size and the evolution of language in the hominins. *Curr. Anthropol.* 34:184–193.

Aiello, L.C. & P. Wheeler. 1995. The expensive tissue hypothesis: The brain and the digestive system in human and primate evolution. *Curr. Anthropol.* 36:199–221.

Arensburg, B., A.M. Tillier, B. Vandermeersch, H. Duday, L.A. Schepartz & Y. Rak. 1989. A Middle Paleolithic human hyoid bone. *Nature* 338:758–760.

Arensburg B., L.A. Schepartz, A.M. Tillier, B. Vandermeersch, & Y. Rak. 1990. A reappraisal of the anatomical basis for speech in Middle Paleolithic hominins. *Amer. Jour. Phys. Anthropol.* 83:137–146.

Asfaw, B., Y. Beyene, G. Suwa, R.C. Walter, T.D. White, G. WoldeGabriel & T. Yemane. 1992. The earliest Acheulean from Konso-Gardula. *Nature* 360:732–735.

Bickerton, D. 1990. *Language and Species*. University of Chicago Press, Chicago.

———. 1995. *Language and Human Behaviour*. UCL Press, London, U.K.

Bunn, H. 1981. Archaeological evidence for meat eating by Plio-Pleistocene hominins from Koobi Fora and Olduvai Gorge. *Nature* 291:574–577.

Byrne, R.W. 1996. Relating brain size to intelligence in primates. Pages 1–8 *in* P.A. Mellars & K.R. Gibson, eds., *Modelling the Early Human Mind*. Macdonald Institute for Archaeological Research, Cambridge, U.K.

Byrne, R.W. & A. Whiten. 1992. Cognitive evolution in primates: Evidence from tactical deception. *Man* 27:609–627.

Cachel, S. & J.W.K. Harris (1995) Ranging patterns, land-use and subsistence in *Homo erectus* from the perspective of evolutionary ecology. Pages 51–66 *in* J.R.F. Bower & S. Sartono, eds., *Evolution and Ecology of* Homo erectus (volume I of the Proceedings of the Pithecanthropus Centennial 1893-1993 Congress) *Pithecanthropus* Centennial Foundation, Leiden University, The Netherlands.

Chase, P.G. & H.L. Dibble. 1987. Paleolithic symbolism: a review of current evidence and interpretations. *Jour. Anthropol. Archaeol.* 6:2632–96.

Clutton-Brock, T.H. & P. Harvey. 1980. Primates, brains, and ecology. *Jour. Zool. London* 190:309–323.

Davidson, I. & W. Noble. 1993. Tools and language in human evolution. Pages 363–398 *in* K.R. Gibson, & T. Ingold, eds., *Tools and Language in Human Evolution*. Cambridge University Press, Cambridge, U.K.

Deacon, T. 1992. The neural circuitry underlying primate calls and human language. Pages 121–162 *in* J. Wind, B. Chiarelli, B. Bichakjian & A. Nocentini, eds. *Language Origin: A Multidisciplinary Approach*. NATO ASI Series - Series D: Behavioural and Social Sciences, vol. 61. Kluwer Academic Publishers, Dordrecht, The Netherlands.

Donald, M. 1991. *Origins of the Modern Mind*. Harvard University Press, Cambridge.

———. 1993. Précis of origins of the modern mind: Three stages in the evolution of culture and cognition. *Behav. Brain Sci.* 16:737–791.

Duchin, L.E. 1990. The evolution of articulate speech: Comparative anatomy of the oral cavity in *Pan* and *Homo*. *Jour. Human Evol.* 19:687–698.

Dunbar, R.I.M. 1988. *Primate Social Systems*, Croom Helm, London, U.K.

———. 1992. Neocortex size as a constraint on group size in primates. *Jour. Hum. Evol.* 22:469–493.

———. 1993. Co-evolution of neocortex size, group size and language in humans. *Behav. Brain Sci.* 16:681–735.

———. 1994. Neocortex size and group size in primates: A test of the hypothesis. *Jour. Hum. Evol.* 28:287–296.

Foley, R. 1987. *Another Unique Species*. Longman Scientific and Technical, London, U.K.

Gibson, K.R. 1986. Cognition, brain size, and the extraction of embedded food resources. Pages 93–105 *in* J.G. Else & P.C. Lee, eds., *Primate Ontogeny, Cognition, and Social Behavior*. Cambridge University Press, Cambridge, U.K.

Gowlett, J.A.J. 1992. Tools — the Palaeolithic record. Pages 350–364 *in* S. Jones, R. Martin & D. Pilbeam, eds. *Cambridge Encyclopaedia of Human Evolution*. Cambridge University Press, Cambridge, U.K.

Hawkes, K., O'Connell, J.F., & Rogers, L. 1997. The behavioral ecology of modern hunter-gatherers, and human evolution. *Trends Ecol. Evol.* 12:29–32.

Hawkes, K., J.F. O'Connell & N.G. Blurton Jones. 1997a. Menopause: Evolutionary causes, fossil and archaeological consequences. *Jour. Hum. Evol.* 32:A8–A9 (abstract).

Hawkes, K., J.F. O'Connell, & N.G. Blurton Jones. 1997b. Hadza women's time allocation, offspring provisioning, and the evolution of long post-menopausal lifespans. *Curr. Anthropol.* 38:551–577.

Hawkes, K., J.F. O'Connell, N.G. Blurton Jones, H. Alvarez, & E.L. Charnov, submitted. Grandmothering and the evolution of human life histories.

Houghton, P. 1993. Neandertal supralaryngeal vocal tract. *Amer. Jour. Phys. Anthropol.* 90:139–146.

Isaac, G.Ll. 1975. Stratigraphy and cultural patterns in East Africa during the middle ranges of Pleistocene time. Pages 495–542 *in* K.W. Butzer & G.Ll. Isaac, eds., *After the Australopithecines*. Mouton Press, The Hague, The Netherlands

Keeley, L. & N. Toth. 1981. Microwear polishes on early stone tools from Koobi Fora, Kenya. *Nature* 295:464.

Key, C. & Aiello, L.C., in press. A prisoner's dilemma model of the evolution of paternal care, *Folia Primatol.*

Krings, M., A. Stone, R.W. Schmitz, H. Krainitzki, M. Stoneking & S. Pääbo. 1997. Neanderthal DNA sequences and the origin of modern humans. *Cell* 90:19–30.

Lieberman, P. 1984. *The Biology and Evolution of Language*. Harvard University Press, Cambridge.

Lieberman, P. 1994. Functional tongues and Neanderthal vocal-tract reconstruction — a reply. *Amer. Jour. Phys. Anthropol.* 95:443–450.

Lieberman, P. & E.S. Crelin. 1971. On the speech of Neanderthal man. *Linguistic Inquiry* 2:203–222.

Lieberman, P., J.T. Laitman, J.S. Reidenberg & P.J. Gannon. 1992. The anatomy, physiology, acoustics and perception of speech: essential elements in analysis of the evolution of human speech. *Jour. Hum. Evol.* 23:447–468.

McCarthy, R.C. & D.E. Lieberman. 1997. Reconstructing vocal tract dimensions from cranial base flexion: an ontogenetic comparison of cranial base angulation in humans and chimpanzees. *Amer. Jour. Phys. Anthropol. Supplement* 24:163–164 (abstract).

McHenry, H.M. 1988. New estimates of body weight in early hominids and their significance to encephalization and megadontia in 'robust' australopithecines. Pages 133–148 *in* F.E. Grine, ed. *Evolutionary History of the 'Robust' Australopithecines*. Aldine de Gruyter, New York.

Mellars, P. 1991. Cognitive changes in the emergence of modern humans. *Camb. Archaeol. Jour.* 1:63–76.

Milo, R.G. & D. Quiatt. 1993. Glottogenesis and anatomically modern *Homo sapiens*: the evidence for and implications of a late origin of vocal language. *Curr. Anthropol.* 34:569–598.

34 AIELLO

Monahan, C.M. 1996. New zooarchaeological date from Bed II, Olduvai Gorge, Tanzania: implications for hominid behavior in the Early Pleistocene. *Jour. Hum. Evol.* 31:93–128.

Nobel, W. & I. Davidson. 1991. The evolutionary emergence of modern human behaviour: Language and its archaeology. *Man* 26:222–253.

Oniko, A. n.d. The mandible and the evolution of human language. Unpublished Masters Thesis. Department of Anthropology, University College London, U.K.

Orwen, Michael J. n.d. An "acoustic-signature" model of early speech evolution. A paper presented at the 1996 Annual Meeting of the Language Origins Society, July 11–15, University of Maryland, Baltimore County.

Parker, S.T. & K.R. Gibson, 1979. A developmental model for the evolution of language and intelligence in early hominids. *Behav. Brain Sci.* 2:367–407.

Pinker, S. 1994. *The Language Instinct.* Penguin Books, London, U.K.

Potts, R., & P. Shipman. 1981. Cutmarks made by stone tools on bones from Olduvai Gorge, Tanzania. *Nature* 291:577–580.

Power, C., C. Arthur, & L.C. Aiello. 1997. On seasonal reproductive synchrony as an evolutionary stable strategy in human evolution. *Curr. Anthropol.* 38:88–91.

Povinelli, D.J. & T.M. Preuss. 1995. Theory of mind: evolutionary history of a cognitive specialization. *Trends Neurosci.* 18:418–424.

Reid, K.E. 1997. Early hominid evolution and ecological change through the African Plio-Pleistocene. *Jour. Hum. Evol.* 32:289–322.

Ridley, M. 1989. The number of males in a primate troop. *Anim. Behav.* 34:1848–1858.

Rogers, M.J. 1997. Early *Homo erectus* land use and future planning: Inferences from lithic discard patterns across a 1.6 million-year-old paleolandscape at East Turkana, Kenya. *Jour. Hum. Evol.* 32:A17–A18.

Ruff, C.B., E. Trinkaus, & T.W. Holliday. 1997. Body mass and encephalization in Pleistocene *Homo. Nature* 387:173–176.

Schepartz, L.A. 1993. Language and modern human origins. *Yearb. Phys. Anthropol.* 36:91–126.

Schmid, P. 1991. The trunk of the australopithecines. Pages 225–234 *in* Y. Coppens and B. Senut, eds., *Origine(s) de la bipédie chez les Hominidés.* Editions du CNRS, Paris, France.

Semendeferi, K. H. Damasio, R. Frank, & G.W. Van Hoesen. 1997. The evolution of the frontal lobes: A volumetric analysis based on three-dimensional reconstructions of magnetic resonance scans of human and ape brains. *Jour. Hum. Evol.* 32:375–388.

Shipman, P. & A. Walker. 1989. The costs of being a predator. *Jour. Hum. Evol.* 18:373–392.

Stanley, S.M. 1992. An ecological theory for the origin of *Homo. Paleobiology* 18: 237–257.

Trivers, R.L. 1972. Parental investment and sexual selection. Pages 136–179 *in* B.J. Cambell, ed., *Sexual Selection and the Descent of Man*, Aldine, Chicago.

White, R. 1982. Rethinking the Middle/Upper Paleolithic transition. *Curr. Anthropol.* 23:169–192.

Walker, A. & R.E. Leakey. 1993. *The Nariokotome* Homo erectus *Skeleton.* Harvard University Press, Cambridge.

Wood, B.A. & L.C. Aiello. in press. Taxonomic and functional implications of mandible-based early hominin body mass predictions. *Amer. Jour. Phys. Anthropol.*

Worden, R. in press. The evolution of language from social intelligence. *In* J. Aitchison, J. Hurford & C. Knight, eds., *Proceedings of the Edinburgh Conference on the Evolution of Human Language.* Cambridge University Press, Cambridge, U.K.

Wynn, T. 1991. Tools, grammar and the archaeology of cognition. *Camb. Archaeol. Jour.* 1:191–206.

Comparative Aspects of Human Brain Evolution: Scaling, Energy Costs and Confounding Variables

Robert D. Martin
Anthropologisches Institut & Museum
Universität Zürich-Irchel
Winterthurerstrasse 190
CH-8057 Zürich, Switzerland

Broad comparisons including at least nonhuman primates and perhaps other mammals yield vital background information for understanding human evolution, not least with respect to the brain. Analyses of many species and characters can reveal general principles applicable to the special case of human evolution and are, indeed, essential for testing of explanations based on simple correlations. Biological systems are complex and a simple association or correlation between any two features will often not reveal a direct causal connection. Interactions with potentially confounding variables must be exhaustively explored in order to establish the criterion of isolation. Multiple allometric scaling analyses provide a useful method for comparative studies, although there are three major practical problems (choice of line-fitting procedure, recognition of grade shifts, appropriate control for degree of phylogenetic relatedness) in addition to the universal problem of confounding variables.

One special example of simple association is the apparent temporal coincidence of features in the fossil record (*e.g.*, between the earliest finds of stone tools and the first evidence of increased brain size) and here the estimation of times of origin is of particular importance. Broad comparative evidence indicates that there has been systematic underestimation of dates of origin in the primate tree, such that widely cited times of divergence among hominids are probably too recent. Combined with mounting evidence of a relatively marked divergence between Neanderthals and modern humans, this has direct relevance for interpretations of the latter stages of hominid evolution. Because these hominids had slightly bigger brains than us, it is automatically assumed that they had comparable capacities. We should, however, consider the implications of the fact that brain expansion in Neanderthals was probably to some extent a parallel development. As part of a general recalibration of times of origin in the primate tree, the inferred time of origin of modern humans must also be pushed back in time, and this has implications for the spread of languages.

Certain human features, including spoken language, are unique and there is no direct comparative evidence. Even here, however, comparisons can provide useful supporting information. Numerous explanations have been proposed to explain the three-fold expansion of human brain size in just a few million years, several in-

volving the development of language, certain aspects of behavior linked to language or a combination thereof. In fact, appropriate analysis of brain size reveals
that brain expansion (relative to body size) was already under way in australopithecines, so there is no temporal association with the first appearance of stone
tools. Further, there is no convincing evidence for a direct link between overall
brain size and any specific behavioral feature in primates generally, although individual parts of the brain may be linked to specific features. Here, brain evolution is
explained in terms of a two-phase model in which the overall size of the brain is
constrained by the resources provided by the mother (maternal energy hypothesis), while the sizes of individual components may be subjected to selection. Possible evidence of specific selection is provided by a strong correlation between the
size of the neocortex and group size, although the potential influence of confounding variables has yet to be fully explored. Hence, concatenation of this correlation
with others to suggest that language evolved as an "inexpensive" substitute for social grooming because of the emergence of large group sizes in hominids must be
treated with great caution.

    This contribution reflects the strongly held conviction that a broad-based com-
parative framework is essential for well-founded interpretations of the biological origins of human language. There are at least two reasons for this. Firstly, comparisons
should be widely spread *across species* to generate a more reliable basis for interpretation of human evolution. In the absence of comparative evidence, it is all too easy to
fall into the trap of special pleading, basing arguments on their individual plausibility
rather than on general principles. Even in cases where we are confronted with features
that are in many ways unique to humans, as is the case with spoken language, interpretations will be more convincing if we can identify underlying biological principles
that have general validity. For instance, if we can succeed in establishing a general relationship across primates (or across mammals generally) between the size of the
brain (or of some specific component of the brain) and a particular form of behavior
relevant to the origin of language, we can be far more confident about any conclusions
that we may draw. Secondly, any analyses should be widely spread *across a spectrum
of characters* for the species compared in order to counter the problem of indirect association between features. In analyses restricted to just two features, it is common to
find a correlation between them, but reliable inference of a causal link requires far
more detailed investigation. If the two features examined initially are actually dependent on a third feature that has not been considered, the secondary association between them may be misinterpreted if considered in isolation.
    A graphic recent example of a confounding variable underlying a simply correla-
tion is provided by an analysis that seemed to indicate a significant correlation between the initial letter of an author's surname and probability of citation in the
literature. Names with initial letters earlier in the alphabet showed a higher citation
rate even after excluding cases in which authors' names were in obvious alphabetical
order (Tregenza 1997). This was interpreted as evidence for a causal link of some
kind, and it was even suggested that a correction factor should be applied when considering citation rates of individual authors. At least one subsequent attempt was
made to provide a causal explanation for the observed correlation (Alexander & Andrews 1997). However, reanalysis indicated that surnames beginning with initials
earlier in the alphabet are simply more common. When this confounding factor was
taken into account, the association between alphabetic order and citation rate was no
longer significant (Shevlin & Davies 1997). In other words, the reanalysis indicated
that authors with initial letters earlier in the alphabet are cited more often primarily
because there are more of them! To quote the authors of that revised analysis: "In or-

der to assume any causal relation, the condition of isolation must be established, that is, the relationship between the two variables exists when isolated from all other confounding variables." Of course, hypotheses concerning causal links should be tested with experiments wherever possible. As direct experiments are ruled out when considering hypotheses concerning evolutionary history, we should at least test our inferences through repeated analyses and confrontation with alternative hypotheses, including as many species and as many features as we can.

Morphologically, humans are quite clearly distinguished from other primates in three major contexts: dentition, locomotor pattern and brain size. These features can be traced through the fossil record. One striking feature is that human brain size is both absolutely and relatively the largest among primates, being some three times bigger (on average) than in our closest zoological relatives the great apes. Of course, humans are equally strikingly distinguished from other mammals by behavioral characteristics, some of which are connected with biological adaptations and may leave traces in the fossil record. For instance, tools manufactured with durable materials can be traced comparatively easily through the fossil record. Other human behavioral peculiarities such as burial of the dead and artistic creations can similarly leave preserved traces, although the first recorded cases occur relatively late in the record and have no obvious link to biological features. Spoken language, a universal and unique feature of modern humans, is both fascinating and tantalizing. In the first place, it clearly combines both biological and cultural components that are universal features of modern humans. There can be little doubt that — as a species-typical feature — humans possess a special adaptation of the central nervous system, which is equipped with a "universal grammar" to develop a specific language prescribed by the cultural environment. This special adaptation is referred to as the "language organ" or "language acquisition device" by Noam Chomsky and as the "language instinct" by Steven Pinker (see his chapter in this volume). There are also specific regions of the brain, notably Broca's area and Wernicke's area, that have long been recognized as having some direct association with language functions. Lateralization, with a concentration of language functions on the left side, is also a typical feature of the human brain. On the other hand, it is relatively difficult to trace any biological feature of language back through time and we are generally obliged to fall back on indirect inference. This being the case, any hypotheses that are advanced must be exhaustively tested before we can be confident that any correlations we may find truly indicate a causal connection.

A key feature linking the morphological and behavioral peculiarities of modern humans is the brain. It is generally believed that the impressive overall size of the human brain must be connected in some way with our wide-ranging behavioral skills, notably including spoken language. Indeed, the connection between our large brain and language may seem to be almost self-evident. In addition, it seems reasonable to expect that certain aspects of the brain that are clearly linked to language, such as lateralization of brain function and enlargement of specific brain areas, may be traceable back through the fossil record. A similar expectation applies to the vocal tract, which is directly involved in the production of human speech.

In this contribution, I shall consider in turn a number of general issues connected with a broad comparative approach to the origins of human language. It is important first to consider the pattern and timing of primate evolution, particularly with respect to the radiation of apes and humans (hominoids). The overall evolutionary tree of the primates provides an essential backdrop for broad consideration of, for example, the brain and its relationship to behavior. Indeed, knowledge of primate phylogeny is a prerequisite for reliable interpretation of comparative evidence. It is also necessary to examine the question of times of origin, as reference to specific "established" dates is becoming increasingly common in the literature. Certain inferences concerning human evolution are based on apparent temporal associations, so errors in inference of dates may lead directly to errors in interpretation of such associations. A close focus on the radiation of the hominoids is then required to establish a reliable starting-point for discussion of early hominid ancestry. There are also certain fundamental issues within the hominid branch of the primate phylogenetic tree. One major point concerns the biological characteristics and relationships of the Neanderthals, considered by some to be no more than a subpopulation of the human species but interpreted by others as a separate species with distinctive adaptations. Having dealt with these general aspects of the phylogenetic tree of primates, attention will be directed to the issue of relative brain size in modern primates in comparison to other mammals. The general relationships that emerge will then be used as a basis for discussing relative brain size in hominid evolution. On this foundation, it will be possible to examine various explanations that have been proposed to account for differences in relative brain size among primate species, notably with respect to evolution of the human brain. Finally, evolution of individual brain parts, particularly the neocortex, and a postulated connection with the development of language will be considered.

The Pattern and Timing of Primate Evolution

Broad comparative treatment of primates of course requires an understanding of their phylogenetic relationships. There is now a general consensus regarding the general pattern of evolutionary relationships among primates, supported for modern species by a substantial body of molecular data (Martin 1990; Purvis 1995). Knowledge of primate phylogeny is needed not only for general background information but also because comparative studies should take into account potentially confounding effects of differential degrees of phylogenetic relatedness between the species compared (Felsenstein 1985; Harvey & Pagel 1991; see later).

For discussion of the origins of language in the context of hominid evolution, the evolutionary divergence between apes and humans is, of course, of special relevance. For the finer relationships among living hominoids there is also a general consensus. It is widely accepted that the gibbons branched away first, followed at a later stage by the orangutans, and that our closest zoological relatives are the African great apes (gorillas and chimpanzees). There is a common tendency to assume that it has now been established beyond reasonable doubt that chimpanzees (bonobos and common chimpanzees) are closer to humans than gorillas. Because of this, many authors simply take chimpanzees as models for discussion of the earliest ancestry of hominids. This, however, is unjustifiable on two counts. Firstly, no modern species should ever be taken as a direct model for an ancestral condition. Although chimpanzees are undoubtedly more primitive than humans in many respects, they are by no means primitive in all respects and inference of the earliest ancestral condition for hominids requires a careful process of character-by-character reconstruction, using a wide range of comparative data. Secondly, despite the fact that most molecular studies indicate a closer relationship between chimpanzees and humans, to the exclusion of gorillas, the evidence is by no means conclusive. The morphological evidence in fact indicates that chimpanzees and gorillas are closer to each other than either is to humans. For the time being, therefore, it is safer to adopt the more cautious view that the relationship between gorillas, chimpanzees and humans is an unresolved trichotomy. Arguments depending on a specific relationship between chimpanzees (or bonobos) and humans must be treated with caution.

An overall knowledge of phylogenetic relationships among primates is also important in another crucial respect, namely for inference of times of origin of individual groups and lineages. Because of the burgeoning number of references to specific times of origin in the literature, notably for dates of divergence between African apes and humans, it is easily forgotten that such dates are very provisional. In the case of molecular data, it is vital to bear in mind a major distinction between the pattern of branching relationships within an inferred tree (its topology) and the assignment of dates to individual branching-points (nodes) in the tree. Whereas the topology of the tree may be based exclusively on analysis of a given set of molecular data and can be determined and tested with increasingly sophisticated techniques, dating of nodes almost always depends upon calibration of the tree using at least one date derived from the fossil record. Only in the case of limited trees for modern human populations has it so far been possible to use certain indications of mutation rates as a basis for inferring dates without reference to external paleontological data. Thus, the reliability of the divergence dates used for almost all molecular trees depends directly on the reliability of calibration dates derived from paleontological evidence (often and regrettably just one calibration date per tree).

As noted previously (Martin 1986, 1990), there is a potentially serious inaccuracy in dates of divergence derived from the fossil record in that it is common practice to equate the geological age of the first known representative of any group or lineage with the actual time of origin. While this may seem to be the only objectively safe approach to the problem, it must be recognized that such dates can only indicate *minimum* times of origin. If the fossil record is very incomplete and patchy, the actual date of origin may be considerably earlier than the first known fossil representative of a group or lineage. Using a very simple calculation, it was estimated that less than 3% of species in the primate phylogenetic tree are currently known from the fossil record and that this low sampling level is likely to lead to a substantial underestimation of divergence times (Martin 1993). It was suggested on this basis that the primates of modern aspect may have originated some 80 million years ago (Mya), rather than about 55 Mya, as is still widely assumed. In the absence of a proper model based on realistic assumptions, the general problem was illustrated with a grossly simplified calculation (uniform rate of increase in number of species over time; uniform survival time of 1 My per species) using a scaled-down tree. Subsequently, Gingerich and Uhen (1994) challenged the interpretation that primates could have originated at such an early date. Using a direct probability calculation based on the simple illustration originally provided (Martin 1993), they concluded that the ancestor of modern primates could not have originated prior to 63 Mya. (Note that this, in itself, is a tacit admission that the date of 55 Mya for the earliest known fossil primate of modern aspect could be increased at least by up to 14.5% in order to obtain the actual time of origin.) Gingerich and Uhen went on to infer that the probability of primates originating 80 Mya was less than five in a billion.

Proper assessment of the problems involved in inferring divergence times from a very patchy primate fossil record necessitates calculations based on a more comprehensive model than that used by Martin (1993) or Gingerich and Uhen (1994). Several obvious complicating factors should be taken into account. Known fossil species tend to be clumped in the phylogenetic tree and therefore cannot be regarded as statistically independent data points for probability calculations. Further, the average body size of primates has tended to increase over time. Because the remains of larger-bodied species are generally more likely to be preserved as fossils and are then more easily detectable, the probability of fossilization and discovery has presumably also increased over time. The shape of the phylogenetic tree will also influence calculations. Rather than increasing uniformly over time [(as assumed in the very simple illustration provided by Martin (1993)], species numbers might conceivably increase rapidly at first and then reach an early maximum or, alternatively, increase very slowly for some considerable time before reaching a maximum. It should also be noted that, regardless of the model tree that is used, underestimation of the time of origin will necessarily lead to underestimation of the expected number of fossil species to be considered in any calculation and hence to underestimation of the date of origin. Finally, the probability of discovery of mammalian fossils is also related to latitude, with a bias towards temperate regions and against tropical regions, so it is necessary to allow for a special development in the course of primate evolution. Modern primates are typically inhabitants of tropical and subtropical forests, now predominantly restricted to the southern continents. At the beginning of the Eocene, primates of modern aspect appeared relatively abruptly in the fossil record of the northern continents and then disappeared equally abruptly at the end of the Eocene. This transitional northward expansion of primates undoubtedly reflects an increase in world temperatures during the Eocene, accompanied by an expansion of tropical and subtropical forests. A striking proportion (approximately 12%) of known fossil primate species are Eocene forms from the northern hemisphere and the sampling density of the primate phylogenetic tree should more properly be calculated separately for fossils occurring in the present geographical area in which living primates occur. In combination, these factors greatly reinforce the likelihood that the origin of primates was markedly earlier than has generally been proposed to date.

Four recent phylogenetic reconstructions using DNA sequence data, all of which took the laudable approach of calibrating the ancestral primate node using external dates, have provided strong and consistent empirical support for an early origin of primates. At the same time, they have provided backing for the proposal that the initial diversification of primates was influenced by continental drift (Martin 1990). In the first study (Janke *et al.* 1994), the complete coding region of the mitochondrial genome of a marsupial (opossum) was compared with that of 6 placental mammals (cow, whale, rat, mouse, seal, human). A phylogenetic tree was inferred from the sequences of eight genes showing approximate constancy of rates of change and calibrated with the widely accepted date of 130 Mya for the divergence between marsupials and placentals (undoubtedly a minimum figure). This calibration indicated the following dates of divergence among placentals: rodents (rat + mouse) *versus* cow, whale, seal and human = 114 ±15 Mya; cow + whale + seal *versus* human (*i.e.,* primates) = 93 ±12 Mya.

In the second study, Hedges, Parker, Sibley, and Kumar (1996) used sequence information for 48 genes of humans, mice and cattle and for a smaller sample of genes for four bird taxa to generate a tree showing divergences between the corresponding orders of mammals and birds. They calibrated their tree by taking a date of 310 Mya for the divergence between birdlike reptiles (diapsids) and mammal-like reptiles (synapsids). This age must itself be a *minimum* date, but it is likely to be reasonably reliable because the reptiles concerned were relatively large-bodied (*i.e.,* more likely to be preserved and discovered as fossils) and are documented from rich fossil sites. On this basis, it was inferred that primates diverged from the other orders of mammals examined at least 90 Mya. The resulting calibration of the tree indicates that the initial radiations of both birds and mammals began during the mid-Cretaceous, coinciding with a period of maximum subdivision of land masses through a combination of continental drift and extensive formation of epicontinental seas.

In a third approach, Arnason, Gullberg, Janke, and Xu (1996) used data for complete mitochondrial DNA sequences to generate a tree showing divergences between various mammal species, including a number of primates. They calibrated their tree by taking a date of 55 Mya for the first known whale (cetacean). This age must similarly be a *minimum* date, but is also likely to be reasonably reliable because cetaceans are relatively large-bodied mammals. The calibration applied by Arnason, Gullberg, Janke, and Xu indicated that primates diverged from other orders of mammals at about 90 Mya, thus confirming the estimate provided by Hedges, Parker, Sibley, and Kumar (1996).

Finally, combined analysis of DNA sequences from three mitochondrial genes and two nuclear genes indicates that adaptive radiation from a specific common ancestor gave rise to a group of African mammals containing golden moles, hyraxes, manatees, elephants, elephant shrews and aardvarks (Springer *et al.* 1997). The results "suggest that the base of this radiation occurred during Africa's window of isolation in the Cretaceous period before land connections were developed with Europe in the early Cenozoic era." The mean divergence time between this African group of mammals and other orders of mammals (including primates) is estimated at about 90 Mya.

Recalibration of the time of origin of primates is of crucial significance because it has spin-off effects for dating of nodes throughout the primate tree, including the date of the split between hominids and African great apes and the estimated time of origin of *Homo sapiens*. It now seems highly likely that hominids originated at an earlier date than has commonly been assumed in recent discussions, and this must be borne in mind when discussing inferred dates of origin for human languages in relation to the fossil record. For instance, if the inferred age of the common ancestor of all modern humans is increased by 50% or more through recalibration, this has radical implications for comparison with known fossil specimens, the archaeological record and inference of temporal relationships between language families.

Some Fundamental Issues in Human Evolution

Much has been written about attempts to define what is meant by the term "human" in an evolutionary context and to pinpoint the emergence of humankind. This is, among other things, reflected in discussions of the emergence of the genus *Homo* in the fossil record. In biological terms, however, it must be accepted that clear definition of the emergence of "humankind" is a futile exercise. Any phylogenetic tree is characterized not only by discontinuities between species, which arise through the process of speciation, but also by continuity along lineages, reflecting direct descent from parent to offspring. Whatever process of speciation one may propose, the fact remains that in any arbitrary subdivision of a continuous line of descent the parents of the first humans must be the last apes in that lineage. Although we can of course list several unique biological features distinguishing modern humans from modern African great apes, those features must have appeared progressively and without interruption over the course of evolutionary time. Further, the well-known phenomenon of mosaic evolution applies to hominid phylogeny just as it does to the evolution of any other group of organisms. The features that now distinguish humans from great apes did not emerge in concert at one particular point in time. Changes in the dentition, locomotor apparatus and relative brain size began early and progressed at different rates, while special features such as the manufacture of durable tools and spoken language are relatively late developments.

Against this background, attempts to define the emergence of human uniqueness at a particular point in the hominid evolutionary tree are doomed to failure. One good example is provided by attempts to recognize a particular brain size (commonly assessed through cranial capacity) as defining the threshold to humanity, the "cerebral rubicon" (Vallois 1954). This threshold was set by Vallois at 800 cc, but was subsequently lowered to 600 cc in the classical paper defining *Homo habilis* (Leakey *et al.* 1964). Such arbitrary definitions, which reflect a belief in a firm connection between brain size and behavioral capacity, are of little value. In the first place, there is an almost twofold variation in cranial capacity within hominoid species generally. In modern humans, for example, cranial capacity can vary between about 1000 cc and 2000 cc. Further, there is a difference between the sexes, reflecting sexual dimorphism in body size. In modern humans, although sexual dimorphism in body size is relatively limited, average cranial capacity is about 10% greater in males than in females. Presumably, some degree of sexual dimorphism in body and brain size was present in early hominids. Thus, if the "cerebral rubicon" is defined on the basis of average brain size, rather than on the relative size of any individual's brain, the average female must have attained human status some tens of thousands of years later than the average male!

Of course, cranial capacity is but one example of the many attempts that have been made to define human uniqueness according to criteria that may or may not be recognizable in the fossil record. Language is clearly a strong potential candidate here. Although there has been a great deal of work on the training of great apes to use sign "language" (see Savage-Rumbaugh 1986 for a review), it is clear that there is a major gulf between the best performance of great apes and human language (Terrace 1979; Sebeok & Umiker-Sebeok 1980; Seidenberg & Pettito 1987). It would therefore be of great benefit if morphological features associated with spoken language could be traced back through the fossil record. There is, for example, the possibility of detecting signs of brain lateralization in fossil hominids. Greater development of the cerebral cortex on one side of the brain (a petalia) can be detected on brain casts and three studies have reported asymmetry in endocasts of fossil hominids (LeMay 1976; Holloway & de Lacoste-Lareymondie 1982; Holloway 1988). In fact, however, some degree of cerebral asymmetry has been reported for great apes (LeMay *et al.* 1982). Further, asymmetry in the lengths of certain sulci indicates that in some Old World monkeys the prefrontal and parietal cortical areas are significantly larger on the left side of the brain (Falk 1978). It has, for example, been demonstrated (contrary to earlier reports) that there is a characteristic difference in size of the Sylvian sulcus between left and right hemispheres in macaques (Falk *et al.* 1986). This external evidence of brain lateralization in macaques links up with demonstration of dominance of the left hemisphere in processing of vocal communication (Heffner & Heffner 1984; see also Falk 1987). Hence, some form of lateralization seems to have been already present in Old World monkeys and apes long before the origin of hominids. Indeed, consistent lateralization in sulcal dimensions has also been found in a New World monkey, the capuchin, although it was not detectable in another neotropical species, the spider monkey (Gilissen 1992). Thus, some kind of externally observable difference between left and right hemispheres is found in several nonhuman primates and certain patterns seem to have arisen independently in at least two separate lineages. Nevertheless, it should be noted that Holloway and de Lacoste-Lareymondie (1982) went beyond the mere recognition of cerebral asymmetry in fossil hominids. They made the point that modern humans and fossil hominids are distinguished from other primates by a *combination* of petalia of the left occipital cortex with petalia of the right frontal cortex. Although individual petalias may occur in nonhuman primates, this particular combination is apparently restricted to hominids.

In any case, caution is needed with respect to interpretations of brain lateralization. It has recently been suggested that this phenomenon may be a secondary consequence of large brain size, with hemispheric specialization arising as a consequence of delay in conduction between the two halves of the brain (Ringo *et al.* 1994). Should this interpretation be borne out, the causal link between brain lateralization and language might not be so direct as has commonly been assumed and the association could (at least in part) be a secondary consequence of the overall size of the brain. The apparent causal link between hemispheric specialization and language may conceivably reflect yet another indirect correlation.

An alternative possibility is that features associated with the vocal tract and speech may be detectable in the fossil record. Humans are once again unique in comparison to all other primates in that there is postnatal descent of the larynx producing a unique configuration of the oral region that is related to the production of various sound components in human speech. There have been suggestions that recognizable features of the cranial base indicate whether descent of the larynx has occurred and that Neanderthal skulls lack these features (Lieberman *et al.* 1972; Laitman *et al.* 1979; Lieberman 1984; Crelin 1987). However, this interpretation has been questioned (Falk 1975; Holloway 1983; Houghton 1993) and a fossilized hyoid bone from a Neanderthal failed to reveal any significant difference from the modern human condition (Arensburg *et al.* 1988). In a modified interpretation, Laitman (1985) linked reorganization of the human larynx to the development of basicranial flexion and traced the beginnings of such flexion back to *Homo erectus*, although it is by no means as pronounced as in *Homo sapiens*. On a different tack altogether, MacLarnon (1993) compared dimensions of the vertebral canal between modern humans and the Nariokotome *Homo erectus* specimen. A unique feature of modern humans in comparison to nonhuman primates is that the thoracic part of the canal is enlarged. The specific thoracic enlargement is not seen in the *Homo erectus* specimen. This difference between *Homo erectus* and *Homo sapiens* could simply be due to adaptation for increased muscular movement or control of the trunk. An alternative possibility, however, is that it is associated with increased muscular control of breathing and hence with the development of speech. This evidence, therefore, might indicate that *Homo erectus* was not capable of speech. In stark contrast, Tobias (1987) has argued that several features of brain casts in *Homo habilis* (marked increase in overall size, pronounced transverse expansion of the cerebrum, inferred presence of Broca's and Wernicke's areas) indicate a "new level of organization in cerebral evolution." On this basis, he specifically suggests that the development of human language began with *Homo habilis*. The search for fossilizable indicators of the emergence of human language continues, but it seems very likely that — as with so many other features of human evolution — the process was a gradual one and that no clear threshold to humanity will be recognizable.

One particular aspect of hominid phylogeny that is of special importance with respect to the origin of language and its potential relationship to the evolution of the brain is the status of the Neanderthals. Although many authors have interpreted the Neanderthals as a subpopulation of the species *Homo sapiens*, accumulating evidence has indicated that they were quite distinctive in many respects and should be regarded as a separate species. Numerous morphological differences separating adult Neanderthals from adult modern humans have been reported (*e.g.*, Rak 1986, 1990; Stringer & Gamble 1993; Hublin *et al.* 1996; Schwartz & Tattersall 1996; Rak *et al.* 1996). Even more significantly, morphological differences have been found to distinguish very young Neanderthals from modern humans of comparable age (*e.g.*, Zollikofer *et al.* 1995, in press), further increasing the likelihood of a clear separation. In the light of this accumulated morphological evidence, recognition of a separate species *Homo neanderthalensis* has increasingly seemed to be justified. This conclusion has now received strong support from an analysis of mitochondrial DNA extracted from the Neanderthal type specimen (Krings *et al.* 1997). There is a marked difference between the Neanderthal DNA and that of modern humans and the time of separation between the two lineages has been estimated at a minimum of 600,000 years ago. It should be emphasized that this is most certainly a minimum figure. In the light of the comments made above about the need for recalibration of the entire phylogenetic tree of primates, it seems quite likely that the time of separation between *Homo sapiens* and *Homo neanderthalensis* may be pushed back to one million years ago or even earlier.

Such a clear separation between *Homo neanderthalensis* and *Homo sapiens* has a number of interesting implications that have been obscured by the long-standing interpretation that Neanderthals are no more than an extreme variant of the modern human condition. Once we have accepted that Neanderthals were a separate species, it is a logical next step to ask how deep the separation goes. Because of a general tendency to equate the human condition with possession of a large brain, a clear distinction between modern humans and Neanderthals (whose average brain size was in fact somewhat greater than in present-day humans) seemed inherently unlikely. However, we should now consider the possibility that expansion of the brain took place in parallel, at least to some extent, during the evolution of Neanderthals and that the shared feature of a large brain size may in fact make Neanderthals seem closer to us than they really are. Indeed, if a major part of the expansion of the Neanderthal brain took place as a parallel phenomenon, we should contemplate the possibility that the internal organization of that brain may have differed in important respects, perhaps including the degree of adaptation for spoken language. As a starting point in examining this intriguing possibility, it would be worthwhile to see whether there are any consistent differences in external morphology of endocranial casts between Neanderthals and modern humans.

Relative Brain Size in Mammals

The brain has always occupied a central place in discussions of human evolution, not least because it is obviously connected in some way with behavior. Assessment of the evolution of the brain is, however, a complex matter. In comparisons between species, it is clear that absolute brain size is not a useful indicator of behavioral capacity. Brain size generally increases with body size such that an elephant, for example, has a brain approximately four times bigger than the human brain. A simple ratio between brain size and body size is also uninformative. The relationship between brain size and body size is curvilinear. As a result, although brain size generally increases with body size, the ratio between brain size and body size progressively declines. In the lesser mouse lemur (*Microcebus*), one of the most primitive living primates, the brain represents 3% of body mass, whereas in humans it represents only 2%.

A practical solution to this problem is provided by allometric analysis, which is based on a simple general scaling model for comparative quantitative studies. This approach is, in essence, relatively straightforward. The relationship between body size (X) and any feature of interest (Y), such as brain size, is taken to conform approximately to a power function of the form: $Y = k \cdot X^a$ (where a is the scaling exponent and k the scaling coefficient). This equation can be converted to a linear relationship through the simple expedient of converting the X and Y values to logarithmic form, yielding the following formula: $\log Y = a \cdot \log X + \log k$. A best-fit line determined for a given data set can be taken as describing the general scaling trend, while deviations of individual species above or below the line (reflected by positive or negative residual values) indicate special adaptations of individual species. The residual values can therefore be taken as an indicator of relative brain size. (It should be noted that, for technical reasons, residual values should be kept in logarithmic form as far as possible. One graphic illustration of the problems that can otherwise arise is provided later.) While it should be noted that estimates of relative brain size differ according to the data base used and the taxonomic level of analysis (Holloway & Post 1982), use of this concept undoubtedly represents a major advance over mere reliance on absolute brain size or on simple ratios to body size.

Although the basic concept underlying allometric analysis is theoretically quite straightforward, there are in practice at least three major problems that largely concern statistical aspects (Figure 1). These issues have been extensively discussed elsewhere and will only be briefly summarized here. Firstly, there is continuing

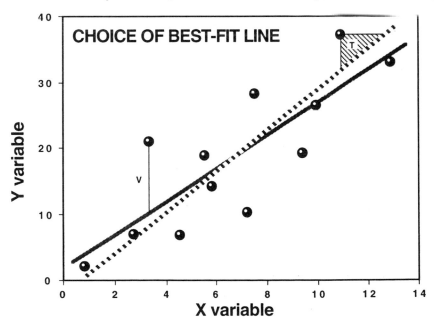

FIGURE 1. Illustration of three fundamental problems in allometric analyses: Problem 1 (above graph): The choice of best-fit line can affect the results of allometric analysis, particularly if there is considerable scatter in the data. In the least-squares regression (continuous line), the sum of the vertical deviations of individual points (*e.g.*, V) is minimized. In this inherently asymmetrical approach, it is assumed that the X variable is independent and free of error. In the reduced major axis (hatched line), the sum of areas of the triangles subtended by individual points (*e.g.*, T) is minimized. In this approach, no *a priori* distinction is made between the variables.

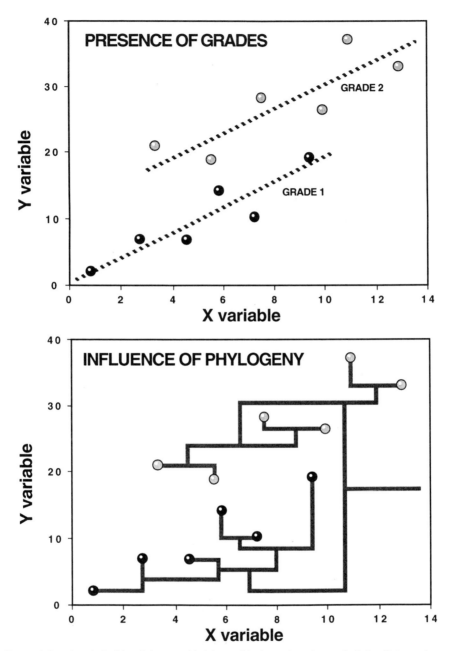

FIGURE 1 (*continued*). Problem 2 (top graph): It is possible that a given data set includes distinct subsets (grades). Commonly, the subsets show similar scaling patterns, reflected by close similarit y in the slopes of the lines (scaling exponent a), but they are separated by a vertical displacement (grade sh ift). Fitting of a single line to a date set containing grades is likely to generate misleading results.

Problem 3 (bottom graph): Statistical testing of scaling differences between species is subject to potential bias due to the differential degrees of phylogenetic relatedness between them.

discussion about the most suitable procedure for determining a best-fit line to describe a scaling relationship. Discussions have mainly revolved around choice between the least-squares regression, the major axis and the reduced major axis (Harvey & Mace 1982; Martin & Barbour 1989). In the analyses reported here, the reduced major axis has generally been taken as the line of best fit, but the use of an alternative procedure would not have affected the results presented. Secondly, it is possible that a given data set may contain subgroups of species, separated by grade differences (Martin 1989a, 1996). If grade differences are present, fitting of a single best-fit line to the data set concerned may yield misleading results. Examples of grade differences are provided in the following text. Finally, it has been suggested that the results of allometric analysis may be biased by differential degrees of phylogenetic relationship between the species included in the sample (Felsenstein, 1985). Felsenstein suggested using "independent contrasts" (differences between successive pairs of taxa in the tree), rather than the raw values, as an appropriate procedure to eliminate the effects of differential degrees of phylogenetic relationship. The basis for this method was subsequently examined in more detail by Harvey and Pagel (Pagel & Harvey 1989; Harvey & Pagel 1991) and the now widely used computer program CAIC was then designed for its application in comparative analyses (Purvis & Rambaut 1995). Contrast analysis using the CAIC program has been applied in some of the analyses reported here as one way of testing for potential biasing effects of phylogenetic relatedness.

At this point, it is essential to note that there is a fourth potential problem that is commonly overlooked: The danger of indirect correlation universally applies to bivariate allometric analyses. A correlation between any two variables, as illustrated in a bivariate plot (*e.g.,* Figure 1), does not necessarily indicate a causal connection between them even if the correlation seems to be very strong. Here, as elsewhere, the criterion of isolation must be respected. It is common to find indirect correlations between variables in bivariate allometric analyses because both are related to one or more additional variables that have not been included in the analysis. For this reason, it is important to conduct extensive analyses in order to test for the presence of indirect correlations. One useful approach here is partial correlation. Using this technique, we can determine whether a correlation between two variables remains after the influence of other potentially confounding variables has been excluded. Successful use of this approach, however, relies upon effective identification of the key interacting variables in any particular analysis.

Having briefly reviewed the major problems involved in scaling analyses, it is now possible to turn to a number of practical applications. When brain size is scaled to body size in a large sample of placental mammals, it emerges that modern humans do, in fact, have the largest relative brain sizes. Examination of residual values for different mammalian orders (Figure 2) reveals that primates are a special case. On average, primates have larger relative brain sizes than members of other mammalian orders. It is, however, important to place this finding in proper perspective. Following the example of many other authors, Dunbar (1992) states that "primates have larger brains … than other animals." Such blanket statements imply that *all* primates have bigger brains than *all* other mammals. This is certainly not true when absolute brain size is considered. As already noted above, the brain of an elephant is some four times bigger than the human brain (the biggest among primates) and several other examples could be cited. It is, however, not even true when the size of the brain relative to body size is considered. After humans, the next highest relative brain sizes among placental mammals are found not in other primates but in dolphins (see Figure 2). Further, there is

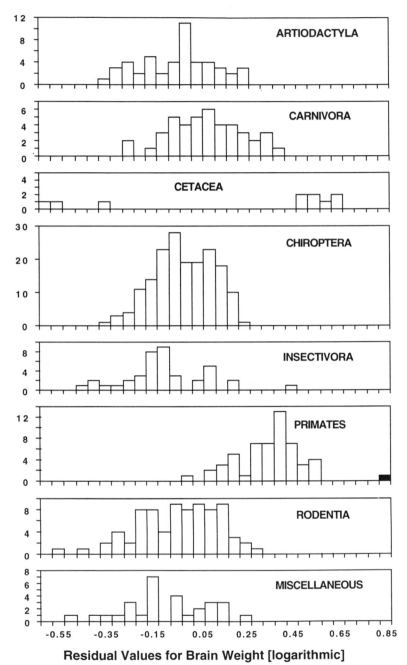

FIGURE 2. Logarithmic residual values for brain size in placental mammals, indicating the size of the brain relative to body size. Primates are clearly a special case in that the values are generally shifted to the right, but there is considerable overlap with other mammals. Humans (indicated in black) have the largest relative brain sizes. The next largest relative brain sizes are found not in other primates but in dolphins, members of the order Cetacea.

considerable overlap between primates and nonprimates in residual values for brain size.

The fact that the *average* value for relative brain size in primates is higher than the average for other mammalian orders (illustrated by the rightward shift of the residual values for primates in Figure 2) can be traced to a difference in neonatal brain size between primates and nonprimates (Figure 3). As a crude approximation, it can be stated that a primate neonate has a brain roughly twice as big as any other neonatal mammal of the same body size. This reflects the fact that, at any given body size, primate fetuses uniformly have larger brains than other mammals throughout development, doubtless because of an early emphasis on brain development in primate embryos (Sacher 1982; Martin 1983). However, because of differences among mammal orders in postnatal development, the marked distinction between primates and nonprimates that is so clearly identifiable at birth becomes partially obscured by the time that adulthood is reached (Figure 2). On the other hand, the fact that the higher average value for relative brain size in primates is connected with a difference in development clearly emphasizes the importance of ontogenetic processes in establishing difference in brain size between species.

So far, this discussion has been confined to the overall size of the brain. It is, in principle, possible that overall brain size reveals little about individual parts of the brain. It turns out, however, that the scaling of individual brain parts in the mammalian brain follows a reasonably consistent pattern. In a wide-ranging study of scaling of individual brain parts in insectivores, primates and bats, Finlay and Darlington (1995) showed that there is a relatively tight association with overall brain size. In other words, it is possible to predict the sizes of individual brain parts from overall brain size to an approximate accuracy of ± 20%. At the same time, it is important to recognize that there is some degree of latitude in the relationships concerned (reflected by scatter of points around the best-fit lines), such that there are differences of detail between species. This indicates that some adjustment of the relationships between individual brain parts does take place, although a basic pattern of brain organization is still recognizable among mammals generally. The study conducted by Finlay and Darlington (1995) was also significant in that it further emphasized the importance of brain development in establishing this basic pattern of mammalian brain organization.

Relative Brain Size in Hominid Evolution

Overall, the fossil record of hominids reveals a progressive increase in absolute brain size over time, although the rate of increase has not been uniform (see Aiello, this volume). Taking four fossil hominid species as generally representative of successive stages, the following sequence in absolute brain size can be documented: *Australopithecus africanus* = 440 cc (n = 7); *Homo habilis* = 630 cc (n = 7); *Homo erectus* = 990 cc (n = 28); modern *Homo sapiens* = 1345 cc (Figure 4). Interestingly, *Homo neanderthalensis* had a larger average brain size than modern humans, with a mean value of 1412 cc (n = 22). Two comments can be made on these numbers. Firstly, it is clear that absolute brain size in hominids has generally increased over a period of at least three million years. Secondly, the average value for *Australopithecus africanus* (440 cc) still lies within the range of average values for great apes, (385 cc for *Pan troglodytes*, 405 cc for *Pongo pygmaeus*, and 496 cc for *Gorilla gorilla*), whereas the

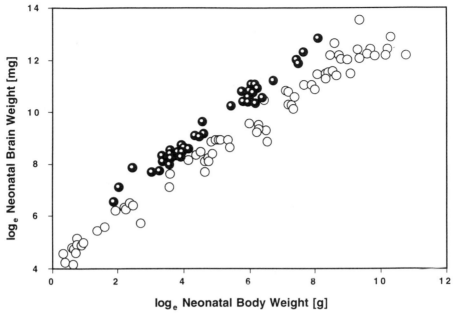

FIGURE 3. Logarithmic plot of brain size against body size for neonates of placental mammals (after Mar -
tin 1996). Primate neonates (dark symbols; n = 43) clearly tend to have larger brains at any giv en body size
than other placental mammal neonates (pale symbols; n = 74). This is a prime example of a distinct grade
shift (see Figure 1b). (Figure reprinted with kind permission from *News in Physiological Sciences*.)

values for all three *Homo* species lie above that level. Because of this, many authors
have concluded that expansion of the hominid brain first began with the genus *Homo*.

As has already been seen, absolute brain size is not very informative across mammals generally and it is therefore necessary to examine relative brain size in fossil
hominids. Here, however, we encounter a problem with respect to the estimation of
body size. Initially, it was believed that all gracile australopithecines, such as *Australopithecus africanus*, were relatively small-bodied with an average body mass of 25-
30 kg. Using this value, Jerison (1973) concluded that relative brain size was, in fact,
greater in *Australopithecus africanus* than in modern great apes. In recent years, however, the consensus view has been that gracile australopithecines showed quite
marked sexual dimorphism and that their average body mass was well above 30 kg.
Jungers (1988), for example, estimated an average body mass of 46 kg for *Australopithecus africanus* using a formula based on apes and humans and an average body
mass of 53 kg using a formula based only apes. Similarly, McHenry (1988) estimated
an average body mass of 46 kg for *Australopithecus africanus* (although he later reported that a value of 36 kg is obtained using a human formula, compared with 46 kg
using an ape formula — see McHenry 1992). If the average cranial capacity of 440 cc
for *Australopithecus africanus* is examined in relation to an average body mass of 46
kg for males and females, the relative brain size of this hominid species is found to fall
within the range of average values for modern great apes. For this reason, it has been
widely concluded that expansion of the hominid brain first began with the genus
Homo even if cranial capacity is considered in relation to body size. Because the earliest reliable evidence for manufacture of stone tools appears in the fossil record at

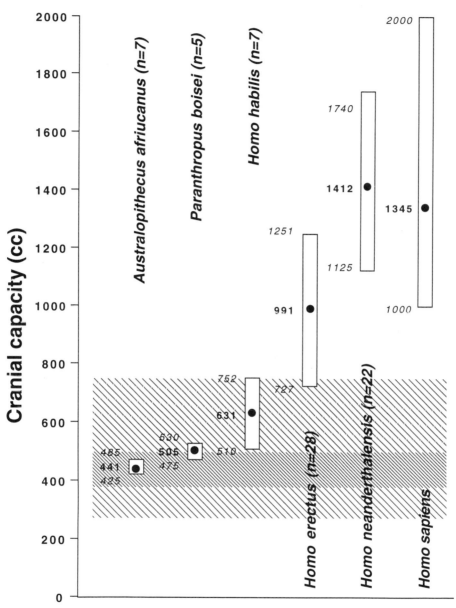

FIGURE 4. Cranial capacities for five fossil hominid species and modern humans. Note the wide range of variation within *Homo* species (mean: value in heavy type opposite black spot; maximum and minimum: values in italics opposite upper and lower ends of white boxes). The hatched zone contains the values for modern great apes (pale hatching: overall range; dark hatching: Range of means for chimpanzee, gorilla and orangutan). The "Cerebral Rubicon" was originally set at 800 cc, above the maximum recorded for great apes, but was later reduced to 600 cc when *Homo habilis* was recognized as a distinct species.

about the same time as the earliest specimens attributable to the genus *Homo*, some authors have concluded that there is a causal connection between tools and the initial increase in relative brain size above the level found in modern great apes. Because it has also been suggested that there is a connection between the mental processes required for manufacture of tools to fit certain design requirements and the mental processes required for language, it might therefore seem that there is some connection between relative brain size in human evolution and language.

There is a major flaw in recent arguments based on revised body mass figures for australopithecines in that all of the values for cranial capacity of *Australopithecus africanus* are derived from skulls that would be interpreted as females by those who believe in the existence of strong sexual dimorphism in this species. The vexed problem of inferring sexual dimorphism in the fossil record can therefore be circumvented by limiting analysis to these "female" gracile australopithecines and female great apes (Martin 1989b). When this is done, it emerges that the cranial capacity of "female" *Australopithecus africanus* relative to body size was in fact some 50% greater than in modern female great apes. This conclusion has recently been broadly confirmed by a study in which body weight was estimated for individual hominid specimens rather than for entire species (Kappelmann 1996).

It is also important here to consider the implications of another widespread fallacy, arising from the implicit notion of "frozen ancestors." If a modern species is taken as a model for an ancestral condition, this implies that the model species itself has remained unchanged over an extensive period of evolutionary time. By taking any modern great ape species as a baseline for comparison with *Australopithecus*, it is inherently implied that the ape's brain size (both absolutely and relatively) has remained unchanged since hominids diverged from the common ancestor. There has, however, been a general trend among mammals for relative brain size to increase in all lineages, albeit at different rates (Martin 1990), so it is likely that brain size has also increased at least to some extent in the lineages leading to modern great apes since they diverged from hominids. Thus, the relative brain size of *Australopithecus africanus* was, if anything, even larger in relation to the common ancestor than the above comparison of female brain sizes has indicated. Overall, therefore, there is a clear implication that the progressive increase in brain size relative to body size during hominid evolution was initiated prior to the first record of *Homo* and prior to the earliest date for recognizable stone tools.

Explanations for Differences in Relative Brain Size

Numerous explanations have been proposed to account for differences in relative brain size among primates. By extension, these may be applied to interpretations of hominid evolution, although a number of additional factors have been invoked for this specific case (*e.g.,* hunting behavior, use and manufacture of tools, language, general "intelligence"). As noted by Dunbar (1992), two basic types of explanation have been invoked to account for differences in relative brain size among primates generally: *Ecological* or *social* explanations. At least three versions of the ecological type of explanation can be identified: (1) frugivores have relatively bigger brains than folivores; (2) relative brain size is associated with the size of the home range; (3) "extractive foraging" favors the evolution of a relatively larger brain. Similarly, at least three versions of the type of explanation invoking social knowledge can be identified, linking relative brain size to: (1) the number of familiar individuals with which social interaction occurs; (2) tracking of social interactions between other individuals; (3) the nature of relationships between individuals. It should be noted that these alternative versions are not necessarily mutually exclusive and that it may be difficult to tease out the main factors involved. For example, the ecological type of explanation is confounded by the fact that both diet and range size are closely associated with group size.

The question of confounding variables is of central importance in the examination of potential links between behavior and relative brain size. In fact, it has been suggested by a number of authors that there may be some connection between an additional factor, metabolism, and brain size (Armstrong 1982, 1983, 1985; Hofman 1983a, 1983b; Martin 1981, 1983). One preliminary indication that there might be such a connection derives from the observation that the value of the scaling exponent (a) is approximately the same (close to 0.75) in the allometric equations relating brain mass and basal metabolic rate to body mass for large samples of mammalian species. Taken alone, this correspondence in the value of the scaling exponent values for brain size and basal metabolic rate does not provide very convincing evidence of a link, although it is suggestive.

Some authors have proposed that the size of the adult brain is directly linked to that individual adult's metabolic capacity. Armstrong (1982) postulated that large brains have high energy demands that "are met by an increase in the energy supply," while Hofman (1983a) suggested that "the energy demands of the brain must be compatible with the oxygen *production* and transport by the body as a whole." It is, however, readily apparent that the connection cannot be such a direct one. For mammals generally, the range of variation in relative brain size is markedly greater than the range of variation in basal metabolic rate relative to body size. Whereas relative brain size shows a fivefold range of variation around the best-fit line (species at the extremes have brains five times as big and a fifth as big as a species lying on the best-fit line), relative metabolic rate shows only a twofold range (species at the extremes have brains twice as big and half as big as a species lying on the best-fit line). Thus, there is a great deal of variation in adult brain size that cannot be explained by a direct relationship with basal metabolic rate of the adults possessing those brains. This is also obvious from examination of the data for primates. As has been shown above (Figure 2), the average value for relative brain size in primates is higher than the average value for any other order of placental mammals. Yet primates do not differ from other orders of placental mammals with respect to the average value for basal metabolic rate relative to body size (Figure 5). Further, the residual value basal metabolic rate in humans does not differ from the average for primates despite the fact that the relative size of the human brain is so outstanding. Accordingly, the higher average value for relative brain size in primates must be attributable to some factor other than a direct connection with basal metabolic rate. It should be noted here that the "expensive tissue hypothesis" proposed by Aiello and Wheeler (1995) is a variant on the theme that the connection between metabolism and brain size is applicable at the level of the individual adult. Their approach differs significantly, however, in invoking a tradeoff between the size of the gut and the size of the brain, as both have relatively high energy requirements. Hence, the size of the gut is a potentially confounding factor that could influence the relationship between brain size and metabolism.

The search for some indirect link between basal metabolic rate and brain size that would also explain a number of other findings (*e.g.*, the difference between primate and nonprimates at birth illustrated in Figure 3) led to formulation of the maternal energy hypothesis (Martin 1981, 1983, 1996). In this, it is proposed that the metabolic turnover of the mother determines the resources available for prenatal development of the brain in the fetus (provided via the placenta) and for postnatal brain development up to the time of weaning (provided via lactation). The brain is relatively unusual compared to other organs of the body in that it reaches its definitive size relatively early in ontogeny, such that a major proportion of brain development has been completed by the time of weaning. In other words, development of the brain is heavily dependent on resources provided by the mother (Figure 6). Thus, the size of the brain in an adult individual may be linked not to that individual's own basal metabolic rate but to the metabolic turnover of its mother. On the one hand, this would account for the general similarity in scaling patterns between brain size and basal metabolic rate relative to body mass (as the values for relative metabolic rate of an adult individual and its mother would be very similar). On the other hand, the greater scatter in residual values for brain size could be attributable to the effects of intervening variables, such as gestation period, lactation period and efficiency of transfer across the placenta and mammary glands. One specific testable prediction that arises from this is that there should be a correlation between gestation period and brain size in addition to any correlation between basal metabolic rate and brain size. The maternal energy hypothesis also differs from other hypotheses in that it could account for the scaling of brain size in the absence of specific selection pressures favoring an increase in the processing capacity of the central nervous system. The potential influence of the maternal contribution to brain development should therefore be considered as one of the factors involved in brain evolution, in addition to any specific selection pressures that might be invoked (Figure 6).

At this point, it is necessary to acknowledge certain challenges that have been made to the maternal energy hypothesis. The first of these concerns a test of the proposed connection between brain size and basal metabolic rate that was conducted by McNab and Eisenberg (1989), with seemingly negative results. This finding has been specifically cited by subsequent authors (*e.g.,* Aiello & Wheeler 1995; Aboitiz 1996) in discussions that omitted any further consideration of the maternal energy hypothesis. For instance, in presenting their "expensive tissue hypothesis" Aiello and Wheeler (1995:211) specifically stated: "These conclusions are derived from the general observation that there is no significant correlation between relative basal metabolic rate and relative brain size in humans and other encephalized mammals."

Quite rightly, McNab and Eisenberg argued that effective demonstration of a link between basal metabolic rate and brain size requires removal of the effect of body size, as this is a potentially confounding variable. It is, in principle, possible that the observed correlation between basal metabolic rate and brain size is an indirect association arising from that fact that both of these variables are correlated with body mass. They analyzed data for 174 mammal species (including monotremes and marsupials) to examine the relationship between relative basal metabolic rate and relative brain size. Although a positive trend was indeed found as predicted, the correlation did not quite reach significance (p = 0.08). It should be noted at once that there is a crucial difference here between hypotheses that invoke some direct link between basal metabolic rate and brain size in the individual adult and the maternal energy hypothesis, which links a mother's metabolism to the completed brain size of her offspring. While it is true that the former predict a very tight association between relative basal metabolic rate and relative brain size, the latter necessarily predicts a weaker association because other variables are involved in the causal chain (Figure 6). Nevertheless, the correlation reported by McNab and Eisenberg is surprisingly weak, even with respect to the maternal energy hypothesis. There was, however, a basic statistical error

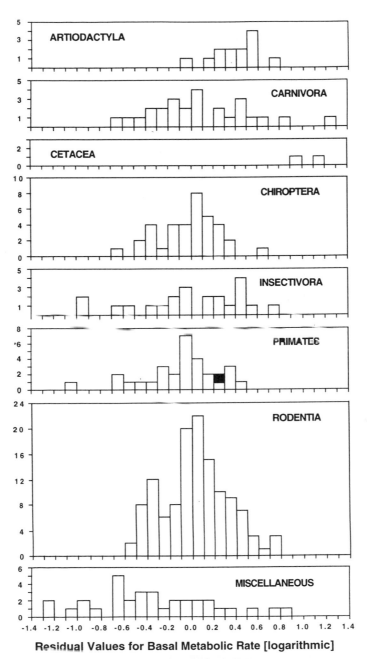

FIGURE 5. Logarithmic residual values for basal metabolic rate in placental mammals, indicating the rate of metabolism relative to body size. Primates, including humans, do not have relatively higher basal meta - bolic rates than other mammals. Further, humans (indicated in black) do not have relatively higher basal metabolic rates than other placental mammals, despite having the largest relative brain siz e. Accordingly, the higher average value for relative brain size in primates (Figure 2) cannot be simply at tributed to a higher average value for basal metabolic rate.

in the analysis conducted. The statistical test used to determine significance was based on the assumption of normality of distribution in the values compared, yet it was applied *after* the logarithmic residual values had been converted to quotients (antilogarithmic form). Because logarithmic residual values are normally distributed, derived quotient values necessarily show a skewed distribution favoring higher values. (For example, the logarithmic residual values for relative brain size in placental mammals are normally distributed around the value of 0 corresponding to species lying directly on the best-fit line. By contrast, derived quotient values for species below the line take values between 0 and 1, whereas values for species above the line take values between 1 and 5.) The appropriate procedure for assessing significance with the derived quotient values is a non-parametric test, such as the Spearman rank correlation, which yields the following result: $r_s = 0.17$; $p = 0.025$. Alternatively, a parametric test (Pearson correlation) can be applied to the logarithmic residual values, yielding the following result: $r = 0.158$; $p = 0.040$. In both cases, the correlation between the residual values for basal metabolic rate and brain size is, in fact, significant. The correlation is not very strong and this reinforces the case for rejecting any direct link in the adult individual between basal metabolic rate and brain size of the kind proposed by Armstrong (1982) and Hofman (1983a, 1983b). Nevertheless, the fact that the correlation is weak but significant (indicating participation of other variables, as

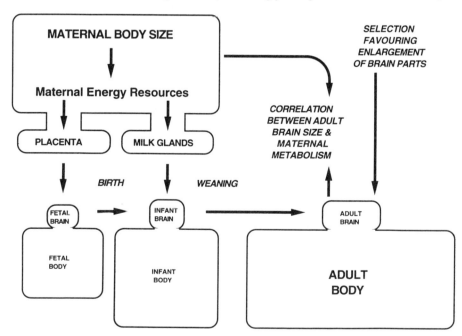

FIGURE 6. Diagram illustrating the maternal energy hypothesis (revised from Martin 1989b). Be cause the brain is unusual in that the major part of its growth occurs early during development, mate rnal resources provided through the placenta and during lactation are particularly important. By the time of weaning, most of the growth in size of the brain has been achieved. Because there is a resulting link be tween a mother's metabolism and the ultimate brain size achieved by her offspring, there will be a secondary cor - relation between that offspring's brain size and its own metabolism once adulthood is reache d. Scaling of maternal resources provides a passive contribution to overall scaling of brain size, whil e individual selec - tion pressures favor the enlargement of particular parts of the brain.

is specifically predicted by the maternal energy hypothesis) should be considered in any overall discussion of the evolution of relative brain size.

Incidentally, given that there is evidence of a connection between basal metabolic rate and total metabolic turnover, it is incorrect to claim that the Aiello/Wheeler hypothesis escapes the requirement for a correlation between residual values for brain size and basal metabolic rate. Consider two species of the same body size, one with a relatively high metabolic rate and one with a relatively low metabolic rate. The species with a relatively higher metabolic rate will be expected to have a larger total energy budget, such that (other things being equal) any "tradeoff" with the digestive tract should leave more energy available to support a large brain. Extrapolation of this simple illustration to a larger sample covering a range of body sizes should surely require a positive correlation between residual values for brain size and basal metabolic rate.

The maternal energy hypothesis has been challenged on two quite different grounds by Pagel and Harvey (1988, 1990). The first relates to the prediction that precocial mammals (those such as primates that give birth to small litters of well-developed offspring) should give birth to neonates with larger brains than altricial mammals (those that give birth to large litters of poorly developed offspring). Pagel and Harvey (1988) stated: "But if species that give birth to precocial offspring also have higher metabolic rates and longer gestations for their size, then Martin's and Hofman's predictions would be supported." This is misleading, as it implies that development of larger brains requires *both* higher metabolic rates *and* longer gestations. It is obvious, however, from the model illustrated in Figure 6 that these two factors can operate independently. Although brain size in the neonate will depend on a combination of maternal basal metabolic rate and gestation period, it is not necessary for both to be elevated in order to produce a large-brained offspring. Indeed, there is evidence that an increase in gestation length may occur in compensation for a relatively low basal metabolic rate (Martin 1996).

The second challenge mounted by Pagel and Harvey is more substantial, as it is argued that some of the findings reported (Martin 1981, 1983) were invalid because of the failure to take litter size into account. This highlights an important issue that requires clarification. Even if the maternal hypothesis is correct in a general sense, there are in fact two different ways in which a mother's energy resources might constrain the development of her offspring's brain. It was initially argued (Martin 1983) that "it is the mother's metabolic turnover which, both in direct terms (through the physiology of gestation) and in indirect terms (through the partitioning of resources between maintenance and reproduction) determines the size of the neonate's brain." At the time, it was unclear to what extent these two aspects of maternal resource allocation explained the findings, but the additional factor of litter size is obviously of great relevance here. If the postulated maternal constraint operates predominantly at the level of partitioning of resources between maintenance and reproduction (*i.e.*, within a life-history framework), then litter size must clearly be taken into account, as an increase in litter size (other things being equal) must increase the total cost to the mother. In that case, however, various other potentially variable factors must also be taken into account. For instance, the interval between births will, of course, have a direct effect on the total cost to the mother, so an increase in litter size could be offset by an increase in interbirth interval. On the other hand, if the maternal constraint is predominantly physiological in kind, the development of the individual fetus may be of prime importance. It can be argued that, regardless of litter size, the development of a fetus depends mainly on maternal metabolic turnover and the length of gestation. Although the presence of competitors within the uterus obviously has some effect, because maternal resources are finite, data for variation in fetal growth according to litter size within a species show that this has a relatively limited effect. Of course, it is impossible to achieve a complete separation between long-term evolutionary effects (*e.g.*, life-history adaptation) and direct physiological effects, as both basal metabolic rate and gestation period have evolved to exhibit particular values for any species. However, given that inclusion of litter size in the analyses yields results conflicting with predictions based on the overall allocation of maternal resources (Pagel & Harvey 1988, 1990), we must consider the possibility that it is the direct physiological constraint that predominates in the relationship between maternal resources and the development of her offspring's brain.

The possibility of direct physiological constraints in the model presented in Figure 6 can be tested with a three-step procedure, using a sample of 51 placental mammal species from 14 different orders for which reliable data are available on body mass, brain mass, basal metabolic rate and gestation period. In the first step, residual values are calculated for brain mass, basal metabolic rate and gestation period relative to body mass. In a second step, residual values for brain size can be examined in relation to residual values for basal metabolic rate, following the example set by McNab and Eisenberg (1989). In fact, the positive correlation that emerges ($r = 0.38$; $r^2 = 0.14$; $p = 0.005$; see Figure 7a) is highly significant and markedly stronger than that found with the data originally reported by McNab and Eisenberg. There could be several reasons for this. The data set used by those authors was very different, notably including two egg-laying monotreme species and 15 marsupial species that are conspicuously different from placental mammals in their reproductive biology. Further, their sample was heavily biased towards rodents (n = 78, representing 45% of the species examined), while only 34 species (20%) were from orders characterized by precocial offspring (artiodactyls, bats, primates). Whatever the explanation may be, the present analysis agrees with that of McNab and Eisenberg (following correction of their analysis as explained above) in showing a significant correlation between relative brain size and relative basal metabolic rate.

Support for the model presented in Figure 6 is, however, even more convincing when the effect of gestation period is included. In the first place, there is a positive and significant correlation between the residuals for brain size and the residuals for gestation period ($r = 0.377$; $r^2 = 0.142$; $p = 0.006$). Further, the model requires that the effects of basal metabolic rate and gestation period should interact. One way of testing this is to examine the relationship between the residuals for brain size and the *sum* of residuals for basal metabolic rate and gestation period. When this is done, there is a marked improvement over the correlation based on basal metabolic rate or gestation period alone ($r = 0.55$; $r^2 = 0.30$; $p\ 0.001$; see Figure 7b). This indicates that basal metabolic rate and gestation period together account for about 30% of the variation in relative brain size between species, which is a very satisfactory result given the other factors that may be involved in brain development. It should be noted, incidentally, that the analyses reported by Pagel and Harvey (1988, 1990) clearly indicated a link between gestation period and brain size; it was the link between brain size and basal metabolic rate that they questioned. Hence, there is good evidence for a link between gestation period and brain size, and the only hypothesis that predicts such a link is the maternal energy hypothesis. An alternative approach, incidentally, is to examine partial correlation coefficients obtained in a four-way analysis of body size, brain size, basal metabolic rate and gestation period. When this is done using the same sample of

51 placental mammal species, it emerges that body size, basal metabolic rate and gestation period influence brain size to approximately equal degrees (Martin, 1996).

There is a potential problem in all of the statistical analyses discussed up to this point, in that the results might be biased by differential degrees of phylogenetic relationship between the species compared (Figure 1). McNab and Eisenberg (1989) took no account of phylogenetic relationship between the species they examined, and it has already been noted above that their sample was heavily biased towards altricial mammals, particularly rodents. Pagel and Harvey (1988, 1990) were well aware of the potential problem of differential phylogenetic relatedness and took steps to eliminate it by conducting their analyses at the level of the family rather than at the level of the species. Although this approach should at least reduce any effect of phylogenetic relatedness, it has a distinct disadvantage in that it drastically reduces sample sizes and may hence dilute or extinguish any signal in the data for this reason alone. In a recent review of the maternal energy hypothesis (Martin, 1996), the possible existence of a bias arising from differential degrees of phylogenetic relatedness was not explicitly examined, for two reasons. Firstly, the sample of 51 mammal species analyzed included representatives from 14 different orders of placental mammals and took only a single species for each genus (thus at least excluding the problem of species-rich genera). Secondly, the method of "independent contrasts," particularly advocated by Harvey and Pagel (1991) and by Purvis and Rambaut (1995) and widely used in recent allometric analyses, is unlikely to work well if numerous marked grade shifts are present in the data. Despite these reservations, the analysis of data for 51 placental mammal species summarized above has been repeated using that method as an additional test. In fact, the correlation between residual values for brain size and residual values for basal metabolic rate (both calculated from their contrasts relative to body mass contrasts) is improved relative to the analysis of the raw data: $r = 0.465$; $r^2 = 0.216$; $p = 0.001$. On the other hand, the correlation between residual contrast values for brain size and residual contrast values for gestation period is reduced relative to the analysis of the raw data and (although remaining positive) becomes nonsignificant: $r = 0.203$; $r^2 = 0.041$; $p = 0.116$. In this case, combining the residual values for gestation period with those for brain size does not improve the correlation with brain size. One interpretation of these results would be that the application of contrast analysis has removed a bias due to phylogenetic relatedness between the species examined and that there is, in fact, no association between relative brain size and the relative length of gestation period. This seems inherently unlikely in view of the results obtained from the analysis conducted at the family level by Pagel and Harvey (1988, 1990), which presumably greatly reduced any bias due to differential phylogenetic relatedness and would at the most be expected to lose correlations because of the dramatic reduction in sample size. Their findings indicated the opposite conclusion, namely that there is a significant correlation between relative brain size and the relative length of gestation but not between relative brain size and relative basal metabolism. An alternative interpretation of the results of the contrast analysis reported here is that the scaling of basal metabolic rate is only mildly affected by grade shifts and that the results therefore survive application of the contrast method, whereas the scaling of gestation period is greatly affected by grade shifts that interfere with the contrast calculations. It is well established that there are major grade shifts in the scaling of mammalian gestation periods, most notably involving a fourfold difference in relative values between altricial and precocial mammals (Martin & MacLarnon 1985). Whatever the explanation may be, it seems clear that there is a significant relationship between relative brain size and relative basal metabolism in the sample examined.

R.D. MARTIN

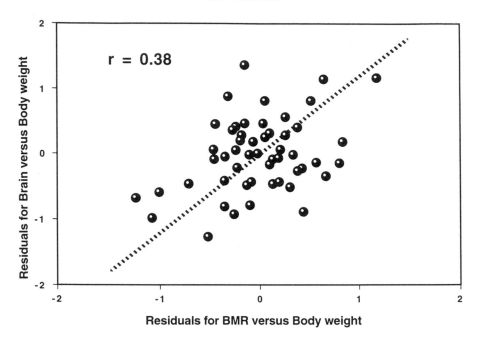

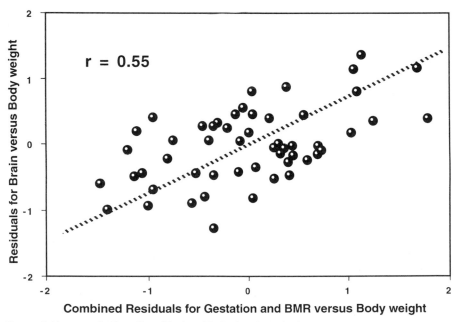

FIGURE 7. Upper graph: Plot of logarithmic residual values for brain size against logarithmic re sidual values for basal metabolic rate for 51 placental mammal species. Although the correlation is highly significant (r = 0.38; p = 0.005), 86% of the variance in brain size remains unexplained. Lower graph: Plot of logarithmic residual values for brain size against combined residual values for basal metabolic rate and gestation period for the same 51 placental mammal species. The correlation is improved by the inclusion of the effect of gestation period (r = 0.55; p 0.001) and the unexplained variance is reduced to 70%.

A number of additional lines of evidence support the inference that maternal resources are of particular importance for the evolution of the brain. For instance, experimental work on genomic imprinting has shown that maternally active genes specifically favor brain development (Keverne *et al.* 1996; Martin 1996). More recently, reexamination of data on the results of human IQ tests has revealed that there is an important contribution of the uterine environment (Devlin *et al.* 1997).

The maternal energy hypothesis addresses the issue of maternal resources required for brain development and the resulting imposition of constraints on overall brain size. It is, however, obvious that selection is likely to influence the size of particular components of the brain, thus ultimately affecting overall brain size. Until recently, it was unclear how the concepts of maternal energy constraints and of selection of individual brain functions could be combined in a single model. A possible connection has now been provided by the two-phase hypothesis of brain size evolution proposed by Aboitiz (1996). His proposal is that brain size is influenced by both "passive" growth (general adjustment to body size) and "active" growth (adaptation to particular behavioral requirements). A strong possibility would seem to be that the maternal energy hypothesis could account (at least in part) for passive adjustment of overall brain size to body size (with the refinement that an increase in maternal metabolic turnover or an increase in the length of gestation, or both factors combined, would also permit an increase in overall brain size), while selection for particular brain functions would eventually translate into an increase in brain size. One corollary of this is that individual behavioral features are unlikely to be reflected more than very indirectly by overall brain size. The search for links between particular behavioral developments, such as language, and increases in brain size should therefore focus particularly on associations between behavior and particular parts of the brain.

Neocortex Size, Group Size and Language

An apt illustration of the advantages and limitations of broad-based comparisons in seeking to explain the origin of human language is provided by analyses examining relationships between individual parts of the brain and a simple measure of social complexity (the typical size of a group of interacting individuals). A prime example is provided by an analysis of the relationship between group size and the volume of the neocortex for 36 primate species conducted by Dunbar (1992). Although there are various problems involved in defining typical group size in a consistent manner across primates, this limitation is probably not severe enough to invalidate the relatively strong correlations that have been determined for some variables. Dunbar reported that, after allowing for the effects of potentially confounding variables such as body mass, there is no significant correlation between the relative size of the neocortex and feeding behavior or ranging behavior (home range size; daily travel distance), but that the relative size of the neocortex does show a significant correlation with group size.

One technical comment is necessary here. Although Dunbar's preferred measure was the "neocortex ratio" (the ratio between the volume of the neocortex and the volume of the rest of the brain), ratios are difficult to interpret because the value can be modified by a change in either the numerator or the denominator, or perhaps both together. Thus, if an increased value of the neocortex ratio is found in any given species, it is not clear to what extent this is due to an increase in the volume of the neocortex as opposed to a decrease in the volume of the rest of the brain. Given that it is the volume of the neocortex (rather than its volumetric relationship with the rest of the brain) which is likely to reflect processing capacity, this variable should be considered in its own right. [See Barton (1993) and Deacon (1993) for comments on additional problems arising from the use of the neocortex ratio.)] In fact, the basic results of Dunbar's original analysis remain largely intact regardless of whether neocortex volume or his neocortex ratio is taken.

In the original analysis of his data, Dunbar did not explicitly take account of potential problems due to differential degrees of phylogenetic relatedness between the species compared, although he did subsequently apply a form of contrast analysis to a subset of his sample (Dunbar 1995). In order to conduct a further check on his findings, his data have been reanalyzed here using the "independent contrasts" method (Purvis & Rambaut 1995). A significant correlation between the residual values for neocortex volume and for group size (*i.e.*, after excluding the influence of body size for both variables) is still found following calculation of contrast values: $r = 0.467$; $r^2 = 0.218$; $p = 0.005$. A very similar result was reported by Barton (1993, 1996), although in his later paper he examined contrast values for the residuals for neocortex volume in relation to group size rather than residuals of group size, arguing that body size has little influence on group size. However, Barton (1996) showed that a significant relationship can only be demonstrated for diurnal monkeys and apes. The relationship for prosimians taken alone is not significant, although this is perhaps attributable to the small sample size.

There seems to be a robust correlation between the size of primate groups and the size of the neocortex, after allowing for the effect of body size, although it cannot be ruled out that additional confounding variables might be found in the future. Indeed, Barton (1996) showed for diurnal monkeys and apes that neocortex size is correlated not only with group size but also independently with degree of frugivory, so social group size is clearly not the only factor linked to the relative size of the neocortex. Here as elsewhere, the criterion of isolation must be firmly established and a great deal of further testing is required before it can be accepted with any confidence that there is a direct causal link between the size of the neocortex and social group size.

The suspicion that there may be far more to this story than initially meets the eye is reinforced by a closer examination of Dunbar's concept of "neocortex ratio." In some analyses at least, this ratio seems to yield better correlations with group size than neocortex volume itself, although it is surely the processing capacity of the neocortex that should be at stake, not its size in relation to the rest of the brain. The higher correlations reported for the neocortex ratio arise because the strong positive correlation between relative group size and relative neocortex volume is matched by an equally strong *negative* correlation between relative group size and the relative size of the rest of the brain. (This results holds regardless of whether the analysis is based on raw values or on contrast values and regardless of whether it is conducted with the entire sample or just with monkeys and apes.) In parallel with the argument that a positive correlation between group size and neocortex volume reflects a causal relationship, one might equally well postulate that increase in brain size is causally related to a reduction in the size of the rest of the brain in primates. One possible explanation might be that there is a tradeoff between the size of the neocortex and the size of the rest of the brain in adaptation to group size. This, in itself, would reinforce the idea that there is some kind of constraint on overall brain size, as suggested by the maternal energy hypothesis. Hence, a much more detailed analysis is required to tease out the causal factors involved.

The identified relationships between the volume of the neocortex and group size or degree of frugivory in any case provide a good potential illustration of the "active" phase of the model suggested by Aboitiz (Figure 8). It can be argued that behavioral requirements associated with group size or diet have served as selections pressure favoring the development of a specific part of the brain, namely the neocortex. By contrast, there is no correlation between group size and other parts of the brain, so selection associated with this variable has not favored a direct increase in brain size as a whole but an indirect increase through enlargement of the neocortex.

In subsequent papers, it has been specifically proposed that the relationship between group size and neocortex volume is directly connected with the evolution of human language (Aiello & Dunbar 1993; Dunbar 1993). Indeed, Aiello and Dunbar (1993) suggested that "the need for large groups among our early ancestors was the driving force behind not only the evolution of language but also hominid encephalization." The chain of argument sets out from the reported significant correlation between group size and neocortex size in nonhuman primates. This empirical bivariate relationship is extrapolated to derive an expected "natural" group size of 150 for humans from the volume of the human neocortex. This inferred group size is then considered in connection with another empirical relationship reported by Dunbar (1991), namely between social grooming time and group size for Old World monkeys and apes. This relationship is interpreted on the basis of the assumption that social grooming is the primary factor in maintaining the cohesion of primate groups and social bonding over time. Taking the inferred human group size of 150, it is predicted (by extrapolation beyond the range of data for Old World monkeys and apes) that such a group size would be expected to spend some 40% time in grooming, whereas 20% seems to be the upper limit for nonhuman primates. On this basis, it is argued that lan-

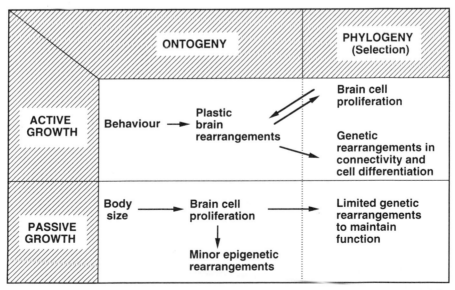

FIGURE 8. Illustration of the two-phase model of brain evolution proposed by Aboitiz (1996). Passive change in brain size is primarily a reflection of body size and it is argued here that maternal resources play a major part in this. Active change in the brain is brought about by selection pressures which lead to enlargement of specific parts of the brain. In the absence of compensatory effects, enlargement of part of the brain will, of course, lead to an increase in overall brain size.

guage evolved as an alternative means of maintaining group cohesion, being more efficient and "cheaper" than grooming and allowing larger mean group sizes. Using estimates of the size of the neocortex from endocranial volumes of fossil hominids, Aiello and Dunbar (1993) went on to infer that some kind of language emerged "early in the evolution of the genus *Homo*."

It should be noted, however, that demonstration of apparent links between social group size, relative size of the neocortex and grooming in nonhuman primates does not necessarily imply a link with language in humans. While it is possible that the development of language is a phenomenon directly associated with the emergence of greater social complexity during human evolution, this is an additional hypothesis that must be adequately tested in its own right.

Acknowledgments

I am very grateful to Nina Jablonski for her invitation to participate in the Third Wattis Symposium and would also like to acknowledge the kindness and efficiency of all those involved in the organization of this event, notably Kathleen Quinlan. The section on calibration of phylogenetic trees profited from valuable discussion with Simon Tavaré, while the sections on allometric scaling greatly benefited from recent discussions with Andrew Barbour, Kate Jones, Ann MacLarnon and Caroline Ross. Andrew Purvis kindly provided a copy of the computer program CAIC, used in some of the analyses reported, and has been very generous with advice on its application. Positive and helpful critical comments from two anonymous reviewers are also gratefully acknowledged. The concept of independent brain size evolution in Neanderthals was prompted by collaboration with Marcia Ponce de León, Christopher Zolloikofer and Peter Stucki in a project on computerized skull reconstruction supported by the Swiss National Science Foundation (projects 3100-032360.91 and 3100-042491.94).

Literature Cited

Aboitiz, F. 1996. Does bigger mean better? Evolutionary determinants of brain size and structure. *Brain Behav. Evol.* 47:225–245.

Aiello, L.C. & R.I.M. Dunbar. 1993. Neocortex size, group size, and the evolution of language. *Curr. Anthropol.* 34:184–193.

Aiello, L.C. & P. Wheeler. 1995. The expensive tissue hypothesis: The brain and the digestive system in human and primate evolution. *Curr. Anthropol.* 36:199–221.

Alexander, J. & J. Andrews. 1997. Alphabets and citations. *Nature* 386:112–113.

Arensburg, B., A.-M. Tillier, B. Vandermeersch, H. Duday, L. Schepartz, & Y. Rak. 1988. A Middle Palaeolithic human hyoid bone. *Nature* 338:758–760.

Armstrong, E. 1982. A look at relative brain size in mammals. *Neurosci. Lett.* 34:101–104.

———. 1983. Relative brain size and metabolism in mammals. *Science* 220:1302–1304.

———. 1985. Relative brain size in monkeys and prosimians. *Amer. Jour. Phys. Anthropol.* 66:263–273.

Arnason, U., A. Gullberg, A. Janke, & X.-F. Xu. 1996 Pattern and timing of evolutionary divergences between hominoids based on analyses of complete mtDNAs. *Jour. Mol. Evol.* 43:650–661.

Barton, R.A. 1993. Independent contrasts analysis of neocortical size and socioecology in primates. *Behav. Brain Sci.* 16:694–695.

———. 1996. Neocortex size and behavioural ecology in primates. *Proc. Roy. Soc. Lond. B* 263:173–177.

Crelin, E.S. 1987. *The Human Vocal Tract.* Vantage, New York.

Deacon, T.W. 1993. Confounded correlations, again. *Behav. Brain Sci.* 16:698–699.

Devlin, B., M. Daniels, & K. Roeder. 1997. The heritability of IQ. *Nature* 388:468–471.

Dunbar, R.I.M. 1991. Functional significance of social grooming in primates. *Folia Primatol.* 57:121–131.

———. 1992. Neocortex size as a constraint on group size in primates. *Jour. Hum. Evol.* 20:469–493.

———. 1993. Coevolution of neocortical size, group size and language in humans. *Behav. Brain Sci.* 16:681–735.

———. 1995. Neocortex size and group size in primates: A test of the hypothesis. *Jour. Hum. Evol.* 28:287–296.

Falk, D. 1975. Comparative anatomy of the larynx in man and the chimpanzee: Implications for language in Neanderthal. *Amer. Jour. Phys. Anthropol.* 43:123–132.

———. 1978. External neuroanatomy of Old World monkeys (Cercopithecoidea). *Contrib. Primatol.* 15:1–95.

———. 1987. Brain lateralization in primates and its evolution. *Yearb. Phys. Anthropol.* 30:107–125.

Falk, D., J. Cheverud, M.W. Vannier, & G.C. Conroy. 1986. Advanced computer graphics technology reveals cortical asymmetry in endocasts of rhesus monkey. *Folia Primatol.* 46:98–103.

Felsenstein, J. 1985. Phylogenies and the comparative method. *Amer. Nat.* 125:1–15.

Finlay, B.L. & R.B. Darlington. 1995. Linked regularities in the development and evolution of mammalian brains. *Science* 268:1578–1584.

Gilissen, E. 1992. Les scissures néocorticales du singe capucin (*Cebus*); mise en évidence d'une asymétrie de la scissure sylvienne et comparaison avec d'autres primates. *C. R. Acad. Sci. Paris, sér. III* 314:165–170.

Gingerich, P.D. & M.D. Uhen. 1994. Time of origin of primates. *Jour. Hum. Evol.* 27:443–445.

Harvey, P.H. & G.M. Mace. 1982. Comparison between taxa and adaptive trends: Problems of methodology. Pages 343–361 *in* King's College Sociobiology Group, ed., *Current Problems in Sociobiology.* Cambridge University Press, Cambridge, U.K.

Harvey, P.H. & M.D. Pagel. 1991. *The Comparative Method in Evolutionary Biology.* Oxford University Press, Oxford, U.K.

Hedges, S.B., P.H. Parker, C.G. Sibley, & S. Kumar. 1996. Continental breakup and the ordinal diversification of birds and mammals. *Nature* 381:226–229.

Heffner, H.E. & R.S. Heffner. 1984. Temporal lobe lesions and perception of species-specific vocalizations by macaques. *Science* 226:75–76.

Hofman, M.A. 1983a. Energy metabolism, brain size and longevity in mammals. *Quart. Rev. Biol.* 58:495–512.

———. 1983b. Evolution of the brain in neonatal and adult placental mammals: A theoretical approach. *Jour. Theor. Biol.* 105:317–322.

Holloway, R.L. 1983. Human palaeontological evidence relevant to language behaviour. *Hum. Neurobiol.* 2:105–114.

———. 1988. Brain. Pages 98–105 *in* I. Tattersall, E. Delson, & J. Van Couvering, eds., *Encyclopedia of Human Evolution and Prehistory.* Garland, New York.

Holloway, R.L. & M.C. de Lacoste-Lareymondie. 1982. Brain endocast asymmetry in pongids and hominids: Some preliminary findings on the palaeontology of cerebral dominance. *Amer. Jour. Phys. Anthropol.* 58:101–110.

Holloway, R.L. & D.G. Post. 1982. The relativity of relative brain measures and hominid mosaic evolution. Pages 57–76 *in* E. Armstrong, & D. Falk, eds., *Primate Brain Evolution*. Plenum Press, New York.

Houghton, P. 1993. Neandertal supralaryngeal vocal tract. *Amer. Jour. Phys. Anthropol.* 90:139–146.

Hublin, J.-J., F. Spoor, M. Braun, F. Zonneveld, & S. Condemi. 1996. A late Neanderthal associated with Upper Palaeolithic artefacts. *Nature* 381:224–226.

Janke, A., G. Feldmaier-Fuchs, W. K. Thomas, A. von Haeseler, & S. Pääbo. 1994. The marsupial mitochondrial genome and the evolution of placental mammals. *Genetics* 137:243–256.

Jerison, H.J. 1973. *Evolution of the Brain and Intelligence*. Academic Press, New York.

Jungers, W.L. 1988. New estimates of body size in australopithecines. Pages 115–125 *in* F.E. Grine, ed., *Evolutionary History of the "Robust" Australopithecines*. Aldine de Gruyter, New York.

Kappelmann, J. 1996. The evolution of body mass and relative brain size in fossil hominids. *Jour. Hum. Evol.* 30:243–276.

Keverne, E.B., F.L. Martel, & C.M. Nevison. 1996. Primate brain evolution: genetic and functional considerations. *Proc. Roy. Soc. Lond. B* 262:689–696.

Krings, M., A. Stone, R.W. Schmitz, H. Krainitzki, M. Stoneking, & S. Pääbo. 1997. Neandertal DNA sequences and the origin of modern humans. *Cell* 90:19–30.

Laitman, J.T. 1985. Evolution of the hominid upper respiratory tract: The fossil evidence. Pages 281–286 *in* P.V. Tobias, ed., *Hominid Evolution: Past, Present and Future*. Alan R. Liss, New York.

Laitman, J.T., R.C. Heimbuch, & E.S. Crelin. 1979. The basicranium of fossil hominids as an indicator of their upper respiratory systems. *Amer. Jour. Phys. Anthropol.* 51:15–34.

Leakey, L.S.B., P.V. Tobias, & J.R. Napier. 1964. A new species of the genus *Homo* from Olduvai Gorge. *Nature* 202:7–9.

LeMay, M. 1976. Morphological cerebral asymmetry of modern man, fossil man and nonhuman primates. *Ann. N. Y. Acad. Sci.* 280:348–366.

LeMay, M., M. Billig, & N. Geschwind. 1982. Asymmetries of the brains and skulls of nonhuman primates. Pages 263–278 *in* E. Armstrong, & D. Falk, eds., *Primate Brain Evolution*. Plenum Press, New York.

Lieberman, P. 1984. *The Biology and Evolution of Language*. Harvard University Press, Cambridge.

Lieberman, R., E.S. Crelin, & D.H. Klatt. 1972. Phonetic ability and related anatomy of the newborn and adult human, Neanderthal man, and the chimpanzee. *Amer. Anthropol.* 74:287–307.

MacLarnon, A.M. 1993. The vertebral canal. Pages 359–390 in A.C. Walker, & R.E.F. Leakey, eds., *The Nariokotome* Homo erectus *Skeleton*. Harvard University Press, Cambridge.

Martin, R.D. 1981. Relative brain size and metabolic rate in terrestrial vertebrates. *Nature* 293:57–60.

———. 1983. *Human Brain Evolution in an Ecological Context (52nd James Arthur Lecture on the Evolution of the Human Brain)*. American Museum of Natural History, New York.

———. 1986. Primates: A definition. Pages 1–31 *in* B.A. Wood, L.B. Martin, & P. Andrews, eds., *Major Topics in Primate and Human Evolution*. Cambridge University Press, Cambridge, U.K.

———. 1989a. Size, shape and evolution. Pages 96–141 *in* Keynes, M., ed., *Evolutionary Studies - A Centenary Celebration of the Life of Julian Huxley*. Eugenics Society, London, U.K.

———. 1989b. Evolution of the brain in early hominids. *Ossa* 14:49–62.

————. 1990. *Primate Origins and Evolution: A Phylogenetic Reconstruction*. Chapman Hall/Princeton University Press, London/New Jersey.

————. 1993. Primate origins: Plugging the gaps. *Nature* 363:223–234.

————. 1996. Scaling of the mammalian brain: the maternal energy hypothesis. *News Physiol. Sci.* 11:149–156.

Martin, R.D. & A.D. Barbour. 1989. Aspects of line-fitting in bivariate allometric analyses. *Folia Primatol.* 53:65–81.

Martin, R.D. & A.M. MacLarnon. 1985. Gestation period, neonatal size and maternal investment in placental mammals. *Nature* 313:220–223.

McHenry, H.M. 1988. New estimates of body weight in early hominids and their significance to encephalization and megadontia in "robust" australopithecines. Pages 133–148 *in* Grine, F.E., ed., *Evolutionary History of the "Robust" Australopithecines*. Aldine de Gruyter, New York.

————. 1992. Body size and proportions in early hominids. *Amer. Jour. Phys. Anthropol.* 87:407–431.

McNab, B.K. & J.F. Eisenberg. 1989. Brain size and its relation to the rate of metabolism in mammals. *Amer. Nat.* 133:157–167.

Pagel, M.D. & P.H. Harvey. 1988. How mammals produce large-brained offspring. *Evolution* 42:948–957.

————. 1989. Comparative methods for examining adaptation in primates depend on evolutionary models. *Folia Primatol.* 53:203–220.

————. 1990. Diversity in the brain size of newborn mammals: Allometry, energetics or life history tactics? *Bioscience* 40:116–122.

Purvis, A. 1995. A composite estimate of primate phylogeny. *Philos. Trans. Roy. Soc. Lond. B* 348:405–421.

Purvis, A. & A. Rambaut. 1995. Comparative analysis by independent contrasts (CAIC): An Apple Macintosh application for analysing comparative data. *CABIOS* 11:247–251.

Rak, Y. 1986. The Neanderthal: A new look at an old face. *Jour. Hum. Evol.* 15:151–164.

————. 1990. On the difference between two pelvises of Mousterian context from the Qafzeh and Kebara caves, Israel. *Amer. Jour. Phys. Anthropol.* 81:323–332.

Rak, Y., W.H. Kimbel, & E. Hovers. 1996. On Neandertal autapomorphies discernible in Neandertal infants: A response to Creed-Miles *Jour. Hum. Evol.* 30:155–158.

Ringo, J.L., R.W. Doty, S. Dmeter, & P.Y. Simard. 1994. Time is of the essence: A conjecture that hemispheric specialization arises from interhemispheric conduction delay. *Cereb. Cortex* 4:331–343.

Sacher, G.A. 1982. The role of brain maturation in the evolution of the primates. Pages 97–112 *in* E. Armstrong & D. Falk, eds., *Primate Brain Evolution*. Plenum Press, New York.

Savage-Rumbaugh, E.S. 1986. *Ape Language: From Conditional Response to Symbol*. Oxford University Press, Oxford, U.K.

Schwartz, J.H. & I. Tattersall, 1996. Significance of some previously unrecognized apomorphies in the nasal region of *Homo neanderthalensis*. *Proc. Natl. Acad. Sci. USA* 93:10852–10854.

Sebeok, T.A. & J. Umiker-Sebeok, eds., 1980. *Speaking of Apes: A Critical Anthology of Two-Way Communication with Man*. Plenum Press, New York.

Seidenberg, M. & L.A. Pettito. 1987. Communication, symbolic communication, and language: Comment on Savage-Rumbaugh, McDonald, Sevcik, Hopkins & Rupert (1986) *Jour. Exp. Psychol.: Gen.* 116:279–287.

Shevlin, M. & M.N.O. Davies. 1997. Alphabetical listing and citation rates. *Nature* 388:14.

Springer, M.S., G.C. Cleven, O. Madsen, W.W. de Jong, V.G. Waddell, H.M. Amrine, & M.J. Stanhope. 1997. Endemic African mammals shake the phylogenetic tree. *Nature* 388:61–64.

Stringer, C. & C. Gamble. 1993. *In Search of the Neanderthals*. Thames & Hudson, London, U.K.

Terrace, H.S. 1979. *Nim: A Chimpanzee Who learned Sign Language*. Eyre Methuen, London, U.K.

Tobias, P.V. 1987. The brain of *Homo habilis*: A new level of organization in cerebral evolution *Jour. Hum. Evol.* 16:741–761.

Tregenza, T. 1997. Darwin a better name than Wallace? *Nature* 385:480.

Vallois, H.V. 1954. La capacité crânienne chez les Primates supérieurs et le 'Rubicon cérébral.' *C. R. Acad. Sci. Paris* 238:1349–1351.

Zollikofer, C.P.E., M.S. Ponce de León, R.D. Martin, & P. Stucki. 1995. Neanderthal computer skulls. *Nature* 375:283–285.

Zollikofer, C.P.E., M.S. Ponce de León, & R.D. Martin. (in press). Computer-assisted skull reconstruction: A bridge between anthropology and medicine. *Evol. Anthropol.*

Organization of Semantic Knowledge and the Origin of Words in the Brain

Alex Martin
National Institute of Mental Health
Laboratory of Brain and Cognition
Building 10 Room 4C-104
10 Center Drive MSC 1366
Bothesda, MD 20892-1366

What does it mean to claim that a nonhuman species has words? Recent evidence from cognitive neuroscience indicates that meaning or semantic information about a particular object is represented as a distributed network of discrete cortical regions. Within this network the features that define an object are stored close to the sensory and motor regions of the brain that were active when information about that object was acquired. These semantic representations are active whenever the object is perceived and when its name is produced or heard. The organization of semantic information parallels the organization of the sensory and motor systems in the primate brain. Evidence of similarities in the way object information is stored in the cerebral cortex of human and nonhuman primates may provide a means for assessing the referential status of nonhuman vocalizations.

Until very recently, our understanding of the organization of language in the brain has come from the study of adult humans with deficits in specific language abilities as a result of focal brain damage. For example, it has been known since the latter half of the 19th century that damage to the posterior region of the left temporal lobe (now referred to as Wernicke's area) can produce impaired speech comprehension, whereas damage to the inferior region of the left frontal cortex (now referred to as Broca's area) can produce impaired speech production. These observations have held-up remarkably well (Figure 1) and during the hundred years following Broca and Wernicke we have learned a great deal about how language is represented in the brain from the study of language-impaired individuals (for an excellent review and synthesis see Caplan 1992).

The recent advent of functional brain imaging technologies (*e.g.,* positron emission tomography, PET; and functional magnetic resonance imaging, fMRI) have ex-

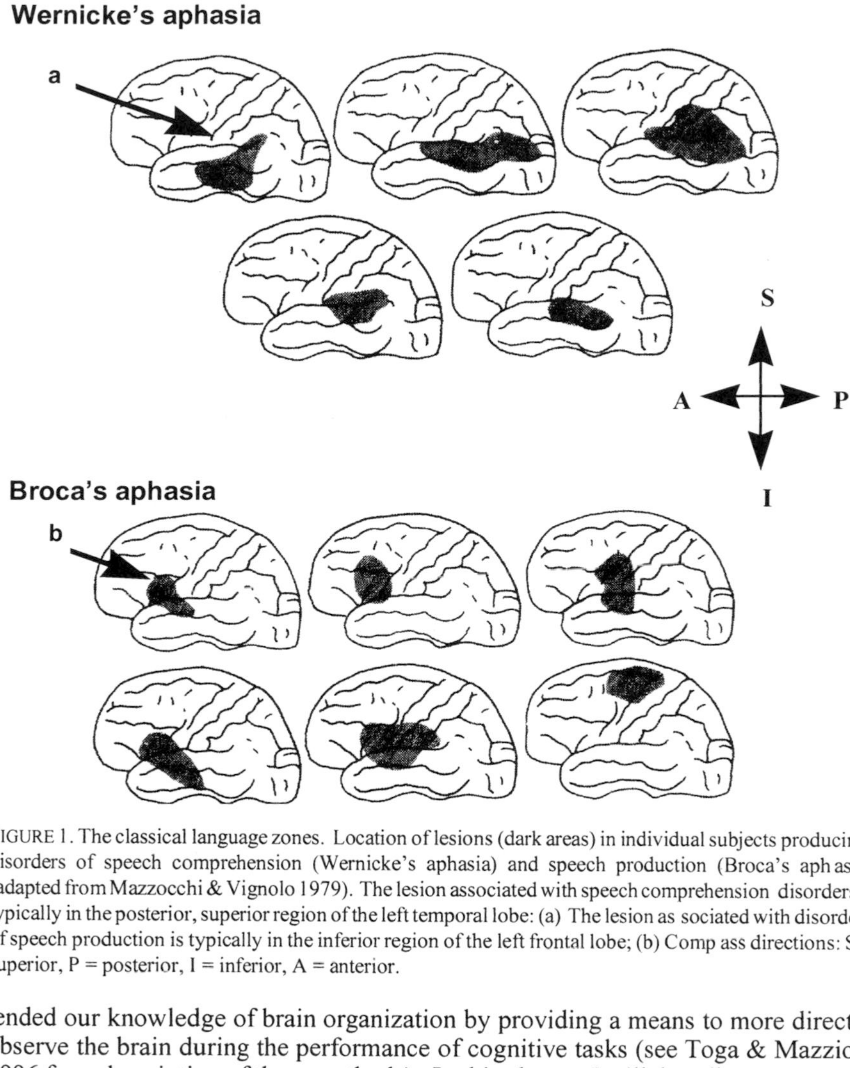

Wernicke's aphasia

Broca's aphasia

FIGURE 1. The classical language zones. Location of lesions (dark areas) in individual subjects producing disorders of speech comprehension (Wernicke's aphasia) and speech production (Broca's aphasia) (adapted from Mazzocchi & Vignolo 1979). The lesion associated with speech comprehension disorders is typically in the posterior, superior region of the left temporal lobe: (a) The lesion associated with disorders of speech production is typically in the inferior region of the left frontal lobe; (b) Comp ass directions: S = superior, P = posterior, I = inferior, A = anterior.

tended our knowledge of brain organization by providing a means to more directly observe the brain during the performance of cognitive tasks (see Toga & Mazziota 1996 for a description of these methods). In this chapter I will describe some recent findings on language processes and brain organization. Rather than focusing on the formal characteristics of language (*i.e.*, word and sentence processing), these studies focus on visual processing of objects as a means of investigating how information about object properties is represented in the brain. The results of these studies suggest a close link between the sites where information about specific features of objects are stored and the sensory and motor systems that were active when that information was acquired. I will then turn to a discussion of these and related findings for understanding the organization of semantic knowledge about concrete objects, and the implication of these findings for understanding the origin of word meaning.

Functionality

Historically, research on language has focused on grammar and syntax, and the apparatus through which language is expressed, namely speech. The available evidence support the view that grammar and speech are singularly human. As a result, focusing on these characteristics of language has served to highlight and to reinforce the discontinuity between man and the rest of the animal kingdom. Grammar, as a rule-based, generative system provides a powerful tool for communication. Given a finite set of rules and tokens (words) an infinite number of meaningful utterances (sentences) can be generated, thereby providing a highly efficient solution or adaptation (Cosmides & Tooby 1995) for solving the problem of intraspecies communication. Nevertheless, we should not lose sight of the fact that language has a function and this function is to communicate meaning, not to generate grammatically correct utterances or to manipulate our vocal cords. What we communicate is our experience of the external world, and our internal world — our images, prelinguistic thoughts, and feelings. These experiences, in turn, are gained through acting in the world (via learned patterns of movement that define our interaction with objects), and through perception (via smell, taste, touch, audition, and especially vision). We, as well as our closest living relatives, are visual animals and the meaning or semantics of things in the world is intimately linked to vision.

As with language, vision also serves a specific function: Building a description, or representation of the shape and position of objects (Marr 1982). Thus vision is primarily about representing what objects look like (their shape, color, texture) and where objects are in relation to ourselves and other objects (their location and movement in space), and language serves to convey these experiences, these representations, to ourselves and others.

Visual Semantics and Words in Monkeys

In a series of groundbreaking studies, Robert Seyfarth and Dorothy Cheney have shown that, in the wild, vervet monkeys emit vocalizations that seem to function as words (Cheney & Seyfarth 1990; Seyfarth & Cheney 1992; Marler, this volume). In support of this claim they showed that these monkeys produced specific vocalizations or alarm calls in response to different predators. One type of call was sounded when a martial eagle flew over head, another call was produced when a leopard was spotted nearby, and a third call was produced in response to a snake. Not only were the calls different, but importantly, other monkeys near enough to hear these calls responded differently depending on which call was heard. For example, Seyfarth and Cheney observed that the monkeys would look up and hide in the bushes when the martial eagle call was heard, climb into nearby trees when the leopard alarm call was heard, and stand on their hind legs and search the nearby grass when the snake alarm was heard. Moreover, these alarm call-specific behaviors were observed in response to taped recordings of the calls even though no predators were present. As Seyfarth and Cheney suggest, the alarm calls functioned as representational or semantic signals (Seyfarth & Cheney 1992) and thus share at least one critical feature with human words: They are referential. The calls refer to or stand for a particular object in the environment, and, based on the behavior of the monkeys that hear the call, they elicit a representation of that object in the mind of others. So, as Seyfarth and Cheney would have it, alarm calls are like words because they are representational.

The jury is still out on whether the alarm calls of monkeys function the same way words function in human language and in the human mind. (Although, see Hauser 1996, for suggestions on a research program that would help to answer this question). The calls have some characteristics in common with human words, but apparently not others (for example, monkeys do not appear to communicate with others with the intention of influencing the mental state of the listener; Seyfarth & Cheney 1992). The issue of whether it is appropriate to consider alarm calls as equivalent to human words in all, or even any, meaningful sense will not be settled here. Rather I would like to address a related question: What does it mean to claim that a word (or in the case of the vervet monkey, an alarm call) is representational? Specifically, what type of processes go on inside the brains of the alarm-call producer and the alarm-call hearer that could allow an arbitrary grouping of sounds to "represent" an object?

Where it is Perceived, it is Learned
Where it is Learned, it is Stored

Accumulating evidence from the fields of cognitive psychology and cognitive neuroscience suggest a number of conditions that may need to be fulfilled in order to give alarm calls representational status.

1) From an information-processing view, object perception is associated with the activation of several qualitatively distinct representations. Chief among these is a perceptual representation based on the object's physical features, and a semantic representation based on previously acquired information about the object (*e.g.*, Humphreys *et al.* 1988; Martin 1992) (Figure 2).

2) The semantic representation consists of information about the features and attributes that define the object. Thus, compared to the perceptual representation, the semantic representation is more abstract, containing information about the class of objects, rather than the specific object being viewed. For the vervet monkey, the semantic representation of the martial eagle might include previously learned information about the shape, color and pattern of motion that characterizes these predators and distinguishes them from other similar objects (*i.e.*, harmless birds). Additionally, the semantic representation would include information about the consequences of confronting this predator, which, in turn, produces fear.

3) Within the brain, the information that defines the semantic representation is not localized in any one place. Rather, it is distributed among a number of areas according to the type of object feature being represented. Information about the color of the eagle is stored separately from information about its form, which in turn is stored separately from information about its pattern of movement.

4) The locations or sites in the brain where object feature information is stored are not distributed arbitrarily. Rather each feature is stored close to the region of the brain that mediates perception of that attribute. For example, information about the color of an object is stored near the area of the brain that mediates perception of color; information about motion is stored near the area that mediates perception of motion.

5) The attributes and features critical for uniquely identifying an object (*i.e.*, to distinguish it from other objects in the same semantic category; from other animals, other tools, other pieces of furniture, *etc.*) are bound together as a result of having ex-

LEXICAL REPRESENTATION

WORDS

kangaroo

SEMANTIC REPRESENTATION

INFORMATION ABOUT FEATURES

(FORM, COLOR ,SIZE, MOTION)

PERCEPTUAL REPRESENTATION

PERCEPTION OF FEATURES

(FORM, COLOR ,SIZE, MOTION)

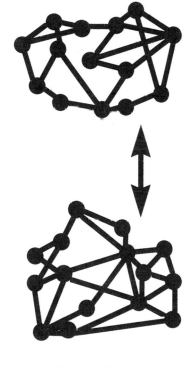

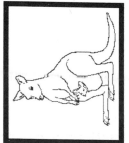

FIGURE 2. Hypothesized neural networks mediating object naming. Perceptual and semantic representations are shown as discrete but interacting networks activated prior to word retrieval.

perienced them together (*i.e.*, they co-occur in time during perception). This binding constitutes a network of discrete cortical regions: a semantic network.

6) This semantic/cortical network is activated automatically (*i.e.*, obligatorily, quickly, and outside of conscious awareness) when an object is viewed. This point becomes evident when we consider that "seeing" as we commonly use the term, refers to "seeing as." To perceive an object is to identify it as a member of some class (*i.e.*, a "dog," "chair," "word," or even a "shapeless form"). Perception, in this everyday usage of the term, cannot occur without the automatic activation of previously acquired information. Typically, for example, it takes less than 700 msec for subjects to name line drawings of common objects, even though the drawings have not been seen previously by the subjects. How could we quickly recognize or identify an object as being of a particular type (*e.g.*, a chair, pencil, or kangaroo) if we did not have prior knowledge of chairs, pencils, and kangaroos?

7) In humans, semantic networks are activated not only when objects are seen, but also when the object's name is read, heard, or retrieved in the service of writing and speech. The name serves as a powerful, economical, shorthand description of just those features that uniquely define the object.

Based on these claims, then, to argue that the alarm calls of the vervet monkey function like words, is to argue that the semantic representation of "martial eagle" is activated not only by perception of the eagle, but also by the sound of the alarm call. This is the critical claim. The alarm call represents the martial eagle because both the perception of the eagle and the alarm call activate a common semantic network in the brain. Presumably, as with the learning of feature-object associations (*i.e.*, learning about the form, color, pattern of motion, *etc.* that define "martial eagle"), the learning of the alarm call-object association may be dependent on the coccurrence of environmental events. In this case, the association between hearing the call and the perception of the eagle, and perhaps also the association between hearing the call and the perception of the call's affect on the behavior of other monkeys.

What is the evidence to support these claims? Before turning to that question it is necessary to briefly describe the organization of the primate visual system.

Organization of the Primate Visual System

The visual system evolved to solve the problem of representing the world. We remain quite far from a formal understanding of how perception is accomplished (*i.e.*, understanding the computations performed in enough detail to build a device that could accomplish the type of simple visual recognition tasks — such as identifying objects from multiple viewpoints — that we accomplish quickly and effortlessly). Nevertheless, we have gained considerable knowledge about the locations and functional properties of the brain regions that mediate vision.

An important starting point for understanding complex brain systems like those that mediate vision is the "principle of modular design" (Simon 1962; Marr 1982). This principle asserts that complex problems are solved by breaking them down into smaller, and presumably more manageable parts. The main idea is that complex systems are composed of subsystems that are as nearly independent of one another as the overall function of the system will allow. If such independence did not exist then even a small change in one part of the system would change the entire system. Thus, in order for evolution to occur in a nonmodular scheme, each change would need to be accompanied by numerous and simultaneous changes throughout the entire system.

Modular design allows for the possibility of modifying or creating new subsystems without necessitating change in all other subsystems.

Until the recent advent of functional neuroimaging in man, the bulk of our knowledge about the modular design of the visual system has come from investigation of one of our closest living relatives, the Old World monkey. Studies of the cortical surface of the macaque have revealed at least 30 separate visual areas occupying nearly one half of monkey cortex (Felleman & Van Essen 1991). These regions are broadly organized into two functional processing streams (Figure 3). An occipitotemporal stream that subserves object vision and an occipitoparietal stream that subserves spatial vision and visual guidance of movements towards objects in space (for recent review see Ungerleider & Haxby 1994). These processing streams are organized hierarchically, with increasingly complex neuronal response properties as one proceeds from primary visual areas in occipital cortex to more anterior sites in the temporal lobe (for the object processing) and parietal lobe (for spatial processing).

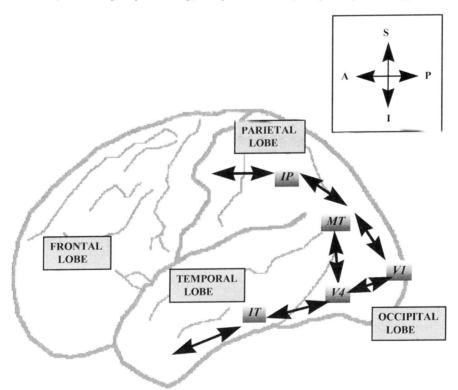

FIGURE 3. Schematic diagram of the two cortical visual systems. Visual information is received in primary visual cortex in the occipital lobe (V1) and then brought forward along two separate processing pathways. An occipitotemporal pathway that mediates object vision (from V1 towards the inferior temporal cortex, IT) and an occipitoparietal pathway that mediates spatial vision (from V1 towards inferior parietal cortex, IP). Each processing stream has extensive feedforward and feedback connections (bidirectional arrows), as well as connections between regions assigned to different processing streams. In the monkey over 30 visual processing regions have been identified, only a few of which are shown here. MT is critical for motion perception and V4 is critical for perception of form and of color (for details see Ungerleider & Haxby 1994).

The need for this separation of function becomes apparent when one considers the work that each system is required to perform. The object recognition system must be designed in such a way as to allow recognition of a particular object as the same object regardless of its position in the visual field. Consistent with this requirement, whereas neurons in the primary visual cortex (in the occipital lobes) have small visual fields, neurons further up stream (in the temporal lobes) have large visual fields (*i.e.*, they respond to a particular object over a large region of space). As a result, information about the exact location of an object is sacrificed in the service of object recognition. While this neural architecture is perfectly suited for visual recognition, it is particularly ill-suited for the job of object localization. Therefore another system, with a different architecture, is needed to keep track of position in space. This job is accomplished by the occipitoparietal spatial processing stream.

Studies of brain-damaged patients have documented a similar organizational scheme in the human brain. For example, damage to the parietal lobes (especially the right parietal lobe) can produce disorders of spatial cognition, including selective deficits in perceiving object location and orientation (Newcombe & Ratcliff 1989), while temporal lobe lesions can produce deficits in object recognition and object naming (especially after left temporal lobe lesions) (Damasio *et al.* 1989).

At a more specific level of analysis, modular design extends to functioning within each processing stream as well. For example, regions in the lower, or inferior aspect of the occipital lobes respond to an object's form and color, whereas other more superiorly located regions respond to an object's direction and speed of movement through space (Desimone & Ungerleider 1989; see Figure 3). Again similar findings have been documented in humans. Damage to the inferior region of the occipital lobe can produce the syndrome of achromatopsia (acquired color blindness; Damasio *et al.* 1980), whereas a more superiorly located lesion at the junction of the occipital, temporal, and parietal lobes can produced akinetopsia (acquired motion blindness; Zeki 1991). Thus, within the cortex, the beginning stages of object recognition are mediated by relatively independent neural modules that subserve perception of specific features of the visual scene. The previously mentioned perceptual representation of an object is mediated by these regions of the brain.

Investigating the Organization of Semantic Attributes

The idea that information about the attributes that define an object may be distributed among different regions of the brain is not new. Wernicke, for example, argued that word forms were stored in one location and received input from visual and other sensory modalities in which modality-specific images of the object concept were stored (as discussed in Head 1926). More recent formulations of the idea that information about different object attributes and features are stored in separate cortical regions has been championed, in somewhat different forms, by Elizabeth Warrington and her colleagues (Warrington & Shallice 1984), Antonio Damasio (1989), and Glynn Humphreys (Humphreys & Riddoch 1987), among others (for review see Saffran & Schwartz 1994; and see Allport 1985 for an influential formulation of distributed semantic representations from a cognitive view). Evidence for this claim, however, has been rather indirect, based almost exclusively on single-case studies of patients with unusual and rare syndromes resulting from focal brain damage and disease.

In order to provide more direct evidence, we set out to investigate semantic representations in the normal human brain using PET (Martin *et al.* 1995). Our working hypothesis was that semantic information about an object is stored as a distributed system in which the attributes that define the object are represented in, or near, the same tissue that is active during perception. Thus, for example, information about the color of an object (*e.g.*, that kangaroos are tan rather than blue) is stored near regions active during color perception, while information about the pattern of motion associated with an object (*e.g.*, that kangaroos hop rather than gallop) is stored near regions active during the perception of motion.

To explore this hypothesis we focused on knowledge about color and motion for two reasons. First, as mentioned previously, lesion studies of both monkeys and humans have shown that perception of color and motion are mediated by separate systems that include distinct regions of the occipital cortex. Moreover, the anatomical location of these regions in man had been identified in earlier PET studies (Corbetta *et al.* 1990; Zeki *et al.* 1991). In addition, studies of patients with focal cortical lesions indicated that retrieval of information about each of these attributes could be selectively disrupted, thus suggesting that semantic information about color and motion also may be stored in separate brain regions. For example, there are reports of patients with selective deficits in naming colors (color anomia; Geschwind & Fusillo 1966) and in retrieving information about an object's typical color (color agnosia, Luzzatti & Davidoff 1994), while other patients have had selective difficulty naming actions associated with the use of an object (*i.e.*, a selective deficit producing action verbs; Caramazza & Hillis 1991; Damasio & Tranel 1993).

The design of our experiments was straightforward. Subjects were shown black and white line-drawings of common objects. During one PET scan they were asked to name the objects, during a second scan they were asked to retrieve the name of a color commonly associated with the objects, and during a third scan they were asked to name an action commonly associated with the objects. For example, in response to an achromatic line drawing of a child's wagon, subjects responded "wagon," "red," and "pull" during the object naming, color word generation, and action word generation conditions, respectively. A second experiment was also run that was identical to the first experiment except that the subjects were presented with the written names of objects, rather than pictures (Martin *et al.* 1995).

Both experiments yielded similar results. Regardless of whether the stimuli were words or pictures, retrieving information about color activated the inferior region of the temporal lobe, just anterior to (in front of) the area known to mediate color perception, whereas retrieving information about action activated a more superior region of the temporal lobe, just anterior to the area known to mediate motion perception (Figure 4).

These results showed that requiring subjects to retrieve previously learned information about object color and motion activated regions of the brain near those that mediate perception of those attributes. This occurred even though the pictures and words presented to the subjects were colorless and motionless. These data thus provided strong evidence for the initial hypothesis: Semantic information about an object appears to be stored as a distributed system in which the attributes that define the object are represented near the same tissue that is active during perception. Most importantly, they suggested that the organization of information storage in the brain follows a similar design as the organization of sensory and perhaps motor systems as well. Information about an object (*e.g.*, a wagon) is not stored as a single entity in a single place. Rather the attributes and features that define the object are stored sepa-

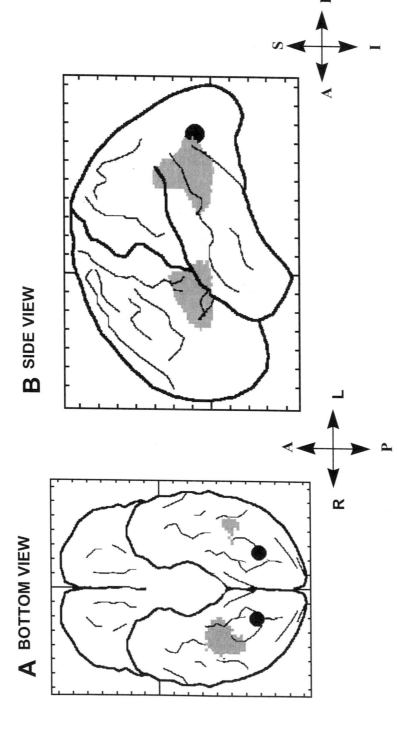

FIGURE 4. (a) Bottom view of the brain showing regions (in gray) more active when subjects retrieved words denoting object-associated colors than when they retrieved words denoting object-associated actions. Black circles show location of areas active when perceiving color. (b) View of the left side of the brain showing regions (in gray) more active when subjects retrieved words denoting object-associated actions than when they retrieved words denoting object-associated colors. Black circles show location of area active when perceiving motion (adapted from Martin et al. 1995). R = right, L = left.

rately. In addition, the sites of storage are near the areas active during the perception of, and therefore when we learned about, those attributes.

More recent work from our laboratory has suggest that brain regions specifically associated with perception are themselves not reactivated when perceptually-based information is retrieved (Chao & Martin submitted). Thus it appears that retrieving information about a specific object attribute like color requires activation of a region of the brain situated close to, but not including, the neural circuitry involved in the perception of color. This finding is consistent with reports of patients with cortical lesions that can no longer see colors, yet retain the ability to imagine colors (Shuren *et al*. 1996), and patients who can no longer see objects, yet retain the ability to imagine objects (Behrmann *et al*. 1992). Taken together, the available evidence suggests that information about object features are stored near, but not in, the tissue active during perception of those features.

Category-Specific Knowledge

The PET studies established three important points with regard to earlier claims about the organization of semantic information. First, retrieving information about different object-associated features is associated with activity in different regions of the brain. Second, the locations of these regions are close to, but do not include, areas associated with the perception of those features. And, third, these regions are active during word retrieval. Retrieving words in appropriate context requires activation of a semantic representation.

To perform these tasks correctly, however, required an appreciable amount of work or effort on the part of the subjects. Specifically, they had to focus attention on previously acquired information about a specific object feature and then find the right word to express that knowledge, all under considerable time pressure (a new stimulus appeared every two seconds). In the model of object recognition sketched previously, however, semantic representations are activated automatically, without effort, whenever an object is seen. Therefore, the next question became: Could we find evidence for the automatic activation of a semantic/cortical network during object identification?

Our strategy for pursuing the answer to this question was the same as the one we used in the color and action knowledge studies. Specifically, we pitted two different categories against each other to determine whether different brain areas became active. This time, however, rather than performing a mentally strenuous and attention-demanding task — retrieving words denoting specific attributes of objects, subjects performed a simpler, less demanding task — naming objects. In fact, for the conditions to be discussed below, subjects were not required to overtly produce names, but merely to view objects and name them silently to themselves.

The categories we chose to study were animals and tools (Martin *et al*. 1996). As with our choice to study knowledge about color and action, this choice of categories was motivated by reports of brain-damaged patients. In this case, reports of patients with selective difficulty naming and answering questions about living things (Warrington & Shallice 1984; Farah *et al*. 1991; Silveri & Gainotti 1988; Sheridan & Humphreys 1993), and reports of patients with deficits limited to man-made objects (Warrington & McCarthy 1983; Warrington & McCarthy 1987; Sacchett & Humphreys 1992).

How could such category-specific impairments occur? One approach to this question has been to deny that these selective deficits actually do occur. This is not an unreasonable position given that category-specific disorders are rare, the between-category dissociation often not pure (*i.e.*, naming may be abnormal for members of both categories, but greater for one than the other), and the findings open to alternative interpretations. In particular, it has been argued that the selective deficit in naming living things is an artifact of differences in the visual complexity of the stimuli used to depict living things and man-made objects (Fennell & Sheridan 1992; Stewart *et al.* 1992). Animals, for example, do tend to have more visually complex forms than tools. As a result, pictures of animals may be more difficult to identify than pictures of tools; especially for a brain-damaged subject. However, such physical differences cannot account for the opposite finding (*i.e., more* difficulty naming man-made than living objects) and recent studies controlling for visual complexity have reduced, if not negated, the explanatory power of the visual-complexity criticism (Farah *et al.* 1996).

Given that category-specific disorders do occur after brain damage, most investigators have relied on some form of a semantic feature model to explain their occurrence. In general, it has been argued that the critical feature used to differentiate members of the category "four-legged animals" is knowledge about physical features. We learn to distinguish animals by their physical characteristics. Moreover, the differences between animals can be quite subtle (consider for example, the difference between horses, donkeys, and mules, or leopards, tigers, and jaguars). Tools, in contrast, while differing in physical form, also have specific functional properties, and these functional properties are the critical component of their definition. This difference in the types of attributes that define animals and tools can be easily verified by consulting a dictionary. This has in fact been done and the results showed that the ratio of physical properties to functional properties is much greater in the dictionary definitions of animals than tools (Farah & McClelland 1991).

This difference in the attributes and features that define animals and tools suggests that the developmental histories of animal and tool learning may differ as well. Knowledge about the unique physical features that define each animal would be acquired primarily through object vision, whereas knowledge about tool differences would be acquired through the motor system (patterns of dominant hand movement learned through the use of tools) and motion vision (patterns of motion learned through observation of tool use by ourselves and others). If these are the kinds of information needed to identify objects, then one would predict that naming animals would require greater activation of previously acquired information about shape or form than would tool naming, whereas tool naming would require activation of information about visual motion and motor movements associated with tool use.

To investigate this hypothesis we asked subjects to silently name briefly presented pictures of objects (Martin *et al.* 1996). Animal pictures were presented during one PET scan and pictures of tools were presented during another PET scan. In addition, subjects were scanned while attending to pictures of nonsense object forms, and while staring at visual noise patterns. Several findings emerged from this study. First, the outer or lateral regions of the left and right occipital lobes were active when subjects perceived objects, regardless of whether they were meaningful (animals and tools) or meaningless (nonsense object forms) (see Malach *et al.* 1995 for a similar finding). This finding suggests that this region of occipital cortex is critical for perceiving object form, and therefore associated with the perceptual, but not the semantic representation of an object (Figure 5). Second, in contrast to nonsense objects,

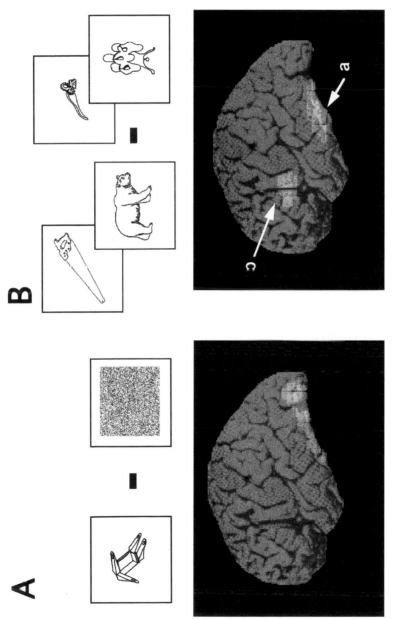

FIGURE 5. A. View of the left side of the brain showing region more active when subjects viewed nonsense objects than when they viewed visual noise patterns. Activation was bilateral, strongest in the occipital lobes, and extended anteriorally into the temporal lobes. B. View of the left side of the brain showing the inferior temporal (a) and inferior frontal regions (b) that were more active when subjects silently named real objects (both animals and tools) than when they viewed nonsense objects (adapted from Martin et al. 1996).

naming meaningful objects (animals and tools) activated the inferior region of the temporal lobes (*i.e.*, a more anterior aspect of the object vision pathway) suggesting that this portion of the temporal lobe may be the site for stored information about object form. Third, naming meaningful objects (animals and tools) activated a region of the inferior frontal lobe known to be associated with speech (Broca's area, Figure 5). Fourth, in addition to areas active when naming both animals and tools, other regions of the brain were selectively activated by naming objects from one category or the other.

In comparison to naming animals, tool naming activated a region of the left temporal lobe that was nearly identical to the region active in the previously discussed studies of action word retrieval (Figure 6). As discussed previously, this region is situated just anterior to (in front of) the area known to be active during motion perception. This finding provides additional evidence that this region of the left temporal lobe may be a critical site for stored information about object motion. In addition, tool naming was associated with activation of a region of the left premotor cortex situated just anterior to the primary motor cortex that controls right-sided body movement (Figure 6). The region of premotor cortex active during tool naming was nearly identical to an area previously found to be active when subjects imagined manipulating objects with their right hand (Decety *et al.* 1994). Thus this region of left premotor cortex may be the site for stored information about patterns of hand movements associated with tool use.

In contrast, the only brain region more active for animal naming than tool naming was on the inner or medial surface of occipital cortex, greater on the left than on the right (Figure 6). This region includes the calcarine cortex which is the first cortical area to receive visual information from the eyes. This finding might be viewed as supporting the idea that category-specific impairments are simply a byproduct of the visual complexity of the pictures, as discussed previously. This explanation, however, was eliminated by the results of a separate study that again found greater medial occipital lobe activity for animal than for tool naming even though the pictures were equated for visual complexity by transforming them into silhouettes (see Martin *et al.* 1996 for details). These results suggest that this early-stage, occipital visual processing area may be reactivated in top-down fashion by regions higher up in the object vision pathway (perhaps via feedback connections from the inferior temporal region associated with identifying meaningful objects). Reactivation of the medial occipital region may be necessary to uniquely identify an object when relatively subtle differences in physical features are the primary means by which the object can be distinguished from other members of its category. Converging evidence for these findings has been provided by a recent study of brain-damaged patients with category-specific naming deficits (Tranel *et al.* 1997).

Object-Associated Affect

The evidence reviewed so far relates to some of the cognitive aspects of object meaning. However, in addition to information about physical and functional features, object meaning can also be emotionally laden. Viewing scenes of accidents, surgical procedures, and the like have an aversive component (and have measurable affects on the autonomic nervous system), whereas pleasant feelings can be elicited by pictures of puppy dogs, flowers, and tranquil environments, *etc*. Moreover, many individuals seems to have an instinctive fear of certain animals (spiders, rats, bats)

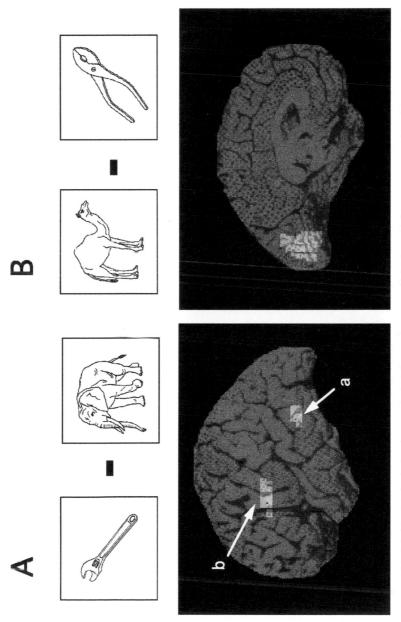

FIGURE 6. A. View of the left side of the brain showing areas in the left posterior temporal lobe: (a) and left premotor cortex (b) and that were more active when subjects silently named pictures of tools than when they silently named pictures of animals. B. View of the inner (medial) surface of the left side of the brain (right side removed) showing the region of the occipital lobe that was more active when subjects silently named pictures of animals than when they silently named pictures of tools (adapted from Martin et al. 1996).

and situations (public speaking, heights) and the negative feelings associated with these experiences can be elicited by viewing pictures. Alarm calls must have an affective component to serve as warnings. In order to function as a warning the sight of a predator (*e.g.*, the martial eagle), and the alarm call that represents it, must elicit an emotional response that signals danger and the appropriate avoidance behavior. Therefore, in addition to feature information, the semantic representation of the martial eagle should include affective information. Similarly, the semantic network activated in the brain of the monkey should include regions that were active when the martial eagle-fear association was established.

Neurobiological studies have established that the amygdala, a structure in the medial region of the anterior temporal lobe, plays a central role in fear conditioning (for a recent review see Ledoux 1996). In addition, studies of patients with lesions confined to the amygdala (*e.g.*, Adolphs *et al.* 1994), and functional brain imaging studies of normal subjects (Breiter *et al.* 1996; Morris *et al.* 1996), provide converging evidence that the amygdala is involved in the visual recognition of emotional expression. For example, in one study (Morris *et al.* 1996) subjects were shown faces and had to decide whether the individual depicted was male or female. The faces depicted different expressions (happy, fear) and varied according to the intensity of expression (ranging from neutral to most fearful or most happy). The data showed that activity in the left amygdala was significantly correlated with the intensity of expressed fear. This occurred even though the task required only gender discrimination, not an emotional response, nor a judgment about emotional expression. This finding is consistent with the idea that the affective valence associated with an object is represented near, if not in, a region critical for learning object-affect associations. Brain regions associated with establishing relationships between objects and emotions may be another component of the semantic network that is automatically engaged whenever an object is seen or its name (or alarm call) heard.

Are Alarm Calls Words?

In this chapter I have described the locations and functions of some of the brain regions that underlie semantic knowledge about concrete objects in humans. What is the relevance of these findings for assessing the referential status of alarm calls in vervet monkeys? Imagine that we could perform a functional brain imaging study of an alert, vervet monkey (such an undertaking would be fraught with technical difficulties; however, we will ignore these problems for the sake of our discussion). One possible outcome would be that the visual presentation of a martial eagle activates a network of cortical regions, and that this same network is activated by the auditory presentation of the martial eagle alarm call (excluding, of course, the primary visual and auditory processing areas associated with the presentation of the object and the call, respectively). Activation of an identical network of brain regions when viewing the predator and hearing the alarm call would provide support for the claim that the alarm call "stands for" the object. That is, we could argue that the object and the call mean the same thing to the monkey *because* they elicit identical states in the monkey's brain.

At the other extreme, there may be no overlap in the regions activated by the object and the alarm call. For example, whereas the visual presentation of the eagle might activate a distributed network of cortical areas associated with stored information about form and motion, the alarm call might activate a limited circuit comprised of auditory cortex and limbic structures associated with learned fear. In this case, the association between the alarm call and the monkey's behavior in the wild would be more like a simple, conditioned fear response (although I think there is good evidence to reject this extreme point of view; see Cheney & Seyfarth 1990). The call would elicit a behavioral response without an intervening stage of cognitive mediation. We could then argue that the call no more "referred" to a martial eagle for the monkey, than the bell referred to a steak for Pavlov's dog.

Concluding Comments: Knowledge Primitives and the Embodied Mind

Writing on the structure of categories, the linguist George Lakoff stated that "Thought is embodied, that is, the structures used to put together our conceptual systems grow out of bodily experience and make sense in terms of it; moreover, the core of our conceptual systems is directly grounded in perception, body movement, and experience of the physical and social order" (Lakoff 1987: xvi). The evidence and arguments presented in this chapter support this view.

The object semantic system discussed here is seen as consisting of learned information about features and attributes that uniquely define an object. This information is represented in the brain as a distributed network of discrete regions in which the attributes that define the object are stored near the regions active when this information was acquired. These include the sensory and motor systems through which we act in, and obtain our experience of, the world. It was further argued that these representations were active not only during object recognition, but during word recognition and production as well. If the alarm calls of the vervet monkeys are referential in the same way as human words, then they would be expected to have semantic representations that follow a similar organizational scheme. Given the similarity between the organization of sensory and motor systems in human and nonhuman primates, the expectation of a similarity in the organization and structure of objects semantics does not seem to be an unreasonable one.

An important remaining question is how do words, and alarm calls, get linked to semantic representations? The idea of coöccurrence of events has limited explanatory power in and of itself because it does not explain why certain events get linked (e.g., words with their referents) and others do not, nor does it explain why this learning happens with ease. Clearly, humans are biologically prepared to establish a link between auditory sounds and object semantics. Perhaps vervet monkeys and other nonhuman primates are prepared to establish such links as well. Nevertheless, humans are prepared to acquire a seemingly unlimited lexicon. The lexical system is both open-ended in capacity and highly flexible in its mapping of words to meaning (i.e., the mapping is many to many). Different words can express the same meaning and the same word can have different meanings. In contrast, the vervet monkey may be prepared to acquire only a limited, genetically determined, lexicon that is closed and rigid in its mappings (one to one).

The type of semantic information discussed in this chapter may be viewed as semantic primitives; as the building blocks out of which more refined shades of meaning could be constructed. The representation of meaning by multiple features stored in different brain regions, rather than as a single entity, provides combinatorial power for representing an infinite number of concepts using a finite number of features. As far as we know, this may be true for both humans and monkeys, but only humans may have the additional capacity to link a multitude of meanings to arbitrary sounds. I have only touched on a few potential candidates for such semantics primitives: knowledge about form, color, motion, action, and affective valence. To this list others could undoubtedly be added, including knowledge of time, space, and number. Although discussion of these semantic features are outside the scope of this chapter, I believe there is evidence from studies of both nonhuman and human primates that point to the existence of localized neural mechanisms that could form the basis for storing information about each of these concepts as well.

Acknowledgments

I thank my colleagues, Leslie Ungerleider, Jim Haxby, Cheri Wiggs, and François Lalonde. I would also like to thank the organizers and sponsors for inviting me to participate in this exciting symposium.

Literature Cited

Adolphs, R., D.Tranel, H.Damasio, & A. Damasio. 1994. Impaired recognition of motion in facial expressions following bilateral damage to human amygdala. *Nature* 372:669–672.

Allport, D.A. 1985. Distributed memory, modular subsystems and dysphasia. Pages 32–61 *in* S.K. Newman & R. Epstein, eds., *Current Perspectives in Dysphasia*. Churchill Livingston, Edinburgh, U.K.

Behrmann, M., G. Winocur, & M. Moscovitch. 1992. Dissociation between mental imagery and object recognition in a brain damaged patient. *Nature* 359:636–637.

Breiter, H.C., N.L. Etcoff, P.J. Whalen, W.A. Kennedy, S.L. Raunch, R.L. Buckner, M.M. Strauss, S.E. Hyman, & B.R. Rosen. 1996. Response and habituation of the human amygdala during visual processing of facial expression. *Neuron* 17:875:887.

Caplan, D. 1992. *Language: Structure, Processing, and Disorders*. MIT Press, Cambridge.

Caramazza, A. & A. E. Hillis. 1991. Lexical organization of nouns and verbs in the brain. *Nature* 349:788–790.

Chao, L.L. & A. Martin. (submitted) Cortical representation of perception, naming, and knowledge of color.

Cheney, L. & R.M. Seyfarth 1990. *How Monkeys See the World: Inside the Mind of Another Species*. University of Chicago Press, Chicago.

Corbetta, M., F.M. Miezin, S. Dobmeyer, G.L. Shulman, & S.E. Petersen. 1990. Attentional modulation of neural processing of shape, color, and velocity in humans. *Science* 248:1556–1559.

Cosmides, L. & J. Tooby. 1995. From function to structure: The role of evolutionary biology and computational theories in cognitive neuroscience. Pages 1199–1210 *in* M.S. Gazzaniga, ed., *The Cognitive Neurosciences*. MIT Press, Cambridge.

Damasio, A.R. & D. Tranel. 1993. Nouns and verbs are retrieved with differently distributed neural systems. *Proc. Natl. Acad. Sci. U.S.A*. 90:4957–4960.

Damasio, A.R. 1989. Time locked multiregional retroactivation: A systems level proposal for the neural substrates of recall and recognition. *Cognition* 33:25–62 .

Damasio, A.R., T. Yamada, H. Damasio, J. Corbett, & J. McKee. 1980. Central achromatopsia: Behavioral, anatomic, and physiologic aspects. *Neurology* 30:1064–1071.

Damasio, A.R., D. Tranel, & H. Damasio. 1989. Disorders of visual recognition. Pages 317–332 in F. Boller & J. Grafman, eds., *Handbook of Neuropsychology vol 2*. Elsevier, Amsterdam, The Netherlands.

Decety, J., D. Perani, M. Jeannerod, V. Bettinardi, B. Tadary, R. Woods, J.C. Mazziotta, & F. Fazio. 1994. Mapping motor representations with positron emission tomography. *Nature* 371:600–602.

Desimone, R. & L.G. Ungerleider. 1989. Neural mechanisms of visual processing in monkeys. Pages 267–299 in F. Boller & J. Grafman, eds., *Handbook of Neuropsychology vol 2*. Elsevier, Amsterdam, The Netherlands.

Farah, M.J. & J.L. McClelland. 1991. A computational model of semantic memory impairment: Modality specificity and emergent category specificity. *Jour. Exp. Psychol.* 120:339–357.

Farah, M.J., M.M. Meyer, & P.A. McMullen. 1996. The living/nonliving dissociation is not an artifact: Giving an a priori implausible hypothesis a strong test. *Cog. Neuropsychol.* 13:137–154.

Farah, M.J., P.A. McMullen, & M.M. Meyer. 1991 Can recognition of living things be selectively impaired? *Neuropsychologia* 29:185–193.

Felleman, D.J. & D.C. Van Essen. 1991. Distributed hierarchical processing in the primate cerebral cortex. *Cereb. Cortex* 1:1–47.

Funnell, E. & J. Sheridan. 1992. Categories of knowledge? Unfamiliar aspects of living and non-living things. *Cog. Neuropsychol.* 9:135–154.

Geschwind, N. & M. Fusillo. 1966. Color naming defects in association with alexia. *Arch. Neurol.* 15.137–146.

Hauser, M.D. 1996. *The Evolution of Communication*. MIT Press, Cambridge, 760 pp.

Head, H. 1963 (first published 1926). *Aphasia and Kindred Disorders of Speech*. Hafner Publishing Company, New York.

Humphreys, G.W. & M.J. Riddoch. 1987. On telling your fruit from vegetables: A consideration of category-specific deficits after brain damage. *Trends Neurosci.* 10:145–148.

Humphreys, G. W., M.J. Riddoch, & P.T. Quinlan. 1988. Cascade processes in picture identification. *Cog. Neuropsychol.* 5:67–103.

Lakoff, G. 1987. *Fire, Women, and Dangerous Things: What Categories Reveal About the Mind*. University of Chicago Press, Chicago.

LeDoux, J. E. 1996. *The Emotional Brain*. Simon & Schuster, New York.

Luzzatti, C. & J. Davidoff. 1994. Impaired retrieval of object color knowledge with preserved color naming. *Neuropychologia* 32:933–950.

Malach, R., J.B. Reppas, R.R. Beson, K.K. Kwong, H. Jiang, W.A. Kennedy, P.J. Ledden, T.J. Brady, B.R. Rosen, & R.B.H. Tootell. 1995. Object-related activity revealed by functional magnetic resonance imaging in human occipital cortex. *Proc. Natl. Acad. Sci. USA* 92:8135–8139.

Marr, D. 1982. *Vision*. W.H. Freeman and Company, San Francisco, California.

Martin, A. 1992. Semantic knowledge in patients with Alzheimer's disease: Evidence for degraded representations. Pages 119-134 in L. Bäckman, ed., *Memory Functions in Dementia*. Elsevier North-Holland, Amsterdam, The Netherlands.

Martin, A., J.V.Haxby, F.M. Lalonde, C.L.Wiggs, & L.G.Ungerleider. 1995. Discrete cortical regions associated with knowledge of color and knowledge of action. *Science* 270:102–105.

Martin, A., C.L. Wiggs, L.G. Ungerleider, & J.V.Haxby. 1996. Neural correlates of category-specific knowledge. *Nature* 379:649–652.

Mazzocchi, F. & L.A. Vignolo. 1979. Localisation of lesions in aphasia: Clinical-CT correlations in stroke patients. *Cortex* 15:627–172.

Morris, J.S., C.D. Frith, D.I. Perrett, D. Rowland, A.W. Young, A.J. Cadler & R.J. Dolan. 1996. A differential neural response in the human amygdala to fearful and happy facial expressions. *Nature* 383: 812–815.

Newcombe, F. & G. Radcliff. 1989. Disorders of Visuospatial Analysis. Pages 333–356 *in* F. Boller, & J. Grafman, eds., *Handbook of Neuropsychology vol 2.* Elsevier, Amsterdam, The Netherlands.

Sacchett, C. & G.W. Humphreys. 1992. Calling a squirrel a squirrel but a canoe a wigwam: A category-specific deficit for artefactual objects and body parts. *Cog. Neuropsychol.* 9:73–86.

Saffran, E. M. & M.F. Schwartz. 1994. Of cabbages and things: Semantic memory from a neuropsychological perspective — a tutorial review. Pages 507–536 *in* C. Umilta & M. Moscovitch, eds., *Attention & Performance XV.* MIT Press, Cambridge.

Seyfarth, R.M. & D.L. Cheney 1992. Meaning and mind in monkeys. *Sci. Amer.* 267:122:128.

Sheridan, J. & G.W. Humphreys. 1993. A verbal-semantic category-specific recognition impairment. *Cog. Neuropsychol.* 10:143–184.

Shuren, J.E., T.G. Brott, B.K.Schefft & W. Houston. 1996. Preserved color imagery in an achromatopsic. *Neuropsychologia* 34:485–489.

Silveri, M.C. & G. Gainotti. 1988. Interaction between vision and language in category-specific semantic impairment. *Cog. Neuropsychol.* 5:677–709.

Simon, H. A. 1962. The architecture of complexity. *Proc. Amer. Philos. Soc.* 106:467–482.

Stewart, F., A.J. Parkin, & N.M. Hunkin. 1992. Naming impairments following recovery from herpes simplex encephalitis: Category specific? *Quart. Jour. Exper. Psychol.* 44A:261-284.

Toga, A.W. & J.C. Mazziotta. 1996. *Brain Mapping: The Methods.* Academic Press, Inc., San Diego, California.

Tranel, D., H. Damasio & A.R. Damasio.1997. A neural basis for the retrieval of conceptual knowledge. *Neuropsychologia* 35:1319–1328.

Ungerleider, L.G. & J.V. Haxby. 1994. 'What' and 'where' in the human brain? *Curr. Opinion Neurobiol.* 4:157–165.

Warrington, E. K. & R. McCarthy. 1983. Category specific access dysphasia. *Brain* 106:859–878.

Warrington, E.K, & T. Shallice. 1984. Category-specific semantic impairments. *Brain* 107:829:854.

Warrington, E.K. & R. McCarthy. 1987. Categories of knowledge: Further fractionation and an attempted integration. *Brain* 110:1273–1296.

Zeki, S. 1991. Cerebral akinetopsia (visual motion blindness). *Brain* 114:811–824.

Zeki, S., J.D.G. Watson, C. J. Lueck, K.J. Friston, C. Kennard, & R.S.J. Frackowiak. 1991. A direct demonstration of functional specialization in human visual cortex. *Jour. Neurosci.* 11:641–649.

Neanderthals, Modern Humans and the Archaeological Evidence for Language

Paul Mellars
Department of Archaeology
University of Cambridge
Downing Street
Cambridge CB2 3DZ, UK

There seems to be widespread agreement that the full panoply of 'Upper Paleolithic' culture in Eurasia, with its rich technology, art, ceremonial and symbolic components, must reflect the presence of essentially 'modern' language patterns, broadly similar to those of present-day populations. The argument is developed here that the behavior associated with the earlier Middle Paleolithic/Neanderthal populations could well reflect a much simpler language structure, of the kind that Bickerton and others have described as 'protolanguage.' Arguably the most relevant features in this context are the apparent absence of explicit 'symbolic' behavior in the archaeological records of the Neanderthals; their apparently simpler patterns of strategic and long-range planning behavior; and simpler and less morphologically structured tool inventories, which may reflect more limited linguistic vocabularies and less 'categorical' forms of mental conceptualization. The much more sharply defined cultural and technological traditions which emerged during the Upper Paleolithic may also be highly significant for the development of language. If these contrasts are accepted, we must presumably look for the origins of essentially modern language in the ancestral African populations, from which the modern populations of *Homo sapiens* apparently emerged. It is argued that some strong indications of this may be discernible in the archaeological records from Africa and southwest Asia between 50,000 and 110,000 years ago. Finally, a critical distinction is drawn between cognitive *potential* and behavioral *expression*, which may help to explain some of the apparent 'anomalies' in the archaeological records of human development over the period of the archaic-to-modern human transition.

Few issues have been more debated recently than the origins of language, and few issues are more problematic (*e.g.*, Parker & Gibson 1990; Bickerton 1990, 1995; Lieberman 1991; Aiello & Dunbar 1993; Gibson & Ingold 1993; Pinker 1994; Aitchison 1996; Dunbar 1996; Noble & Davidson 1996, *etc.*). The problems are obvious. First, what do we mean by 'language' — which is now generally seen as an extremely complex and multifaceted communication system, different elements of which could well have emerged at different points in human evolution, conceivably in response to different environmental and social stimuli? What *were* the kinds of stimuli which provided the essential selective pressures for the evolution of language at different stages in our primate and early human past? Indeed, how far *is* language a biologically and genetically programmed component of our behavior (in Pinker's [1994] terms, a 'language instinct') as opposed to a basic element of 'cultural technology' which emerged at some point (or points) as part of the broader patterns of cultural and technological evolution? Finally, what possible sources of behavioral evidence — as reflected in the archaeological records of human behavior — can we invoke to attempt to document the origins and emergence of language? In other words, what exactly are the likely behavioral and archaeological correlates of varying levels of complexity of language in different behavioral spheres?

The complexity and intransigence of these issues are, to put it mildly, daunting. My own instinct in these situations is to move from the known to the unknown, much as one might tackle a complicated jigsaw puzzle. In other words I prefer to start at the point where no one would seriously question that complex, essentially modern language patterns must have existed, and then to consider what precedes this.

For reasons I hope will become apparent as the paper proceeds a convenient point at which to begin the discussion is at the time of the apparent replacement of the 'archaic' Neanderthal populations of Europe by new and apparently intrusive populations of anatomically modern humans (Stringer & McKie 1996; Stringer & Gamble 1993; Mellars 1996a). This will allow us to focus on a number of critical features of the behavioral and associated archaeological aspects of this transition which I will argue may have a direct bearing on the nature and complexity of language, and may provide some of the key clues as to how specific aspects of archaeological data may relate to specific aspects of language development. In the later part of the discussion I will look at some of the possible implications of this evidence for the earlier stages of language development.

The Human Revolution in Europe

In Europe the period centered on 35–40,000 BP (in conventional radiocarbon terms) witnessed two dramatic changes. On the one hand there was the effective replacement of the earlier, archaic Neanderthal populations which had occupied the continent for at least the previous 200,000 years by populations of physically or anatomically modern humans, closely similar in most anatomical respects to ourselves (Stringer & McKie 1996; Stringer & Gamble 1993; Krings *et al.* 1997). And on the other hand there was a range of conspicuous changes in the archaeological records of human behavior which collectively define the transition from the Middle Paleolithic (or 'Mousterian') to the Upper Paleolithic periods (see Table 1: Mellars 1973, 1989a, 1989b, 1991, 1996a; Farizy 1990; Knecht *et al.* 1993). This transition took place at a point approximately midway during the last glacial period at a time when the more northerly parts of Europe, together with the Alps, the Pyrenees and other more localized mountainous areas were covered by substantial ice caps. Temperatures over this period were oscillatory but for much of the time were probably between 5°C and 10°C lower than those of the present day (Van Andel & Tzedakis 1996). Landscapes over large areas of Europe were dominated by predominantly open tundra or steppe-like vegetation, supporting large herds of reindeer, horse, bison and, in some areas, mam-

TABLE 1. Principal archaeological features of the 'Upper Paleolithic Revolution' in Europe.

1. New 'punch' blade and bladelet technology
2. New forms of stone tools
3. More imposed form in tool manufacture
4. Rapid changes in tool forms
5. Complex, shaped, bone/antler/ivory artifacts
6. Personal ornaments (beads, perforated teeth, *etc.*)
7. Incised/decorated bonework
8. Representational art
9. Long-distance transport of marine shells
10. Musical instruments
11. Increased population size?
12. Increased social group size?
13. More 'structured' occupation sites
14. More specialized, strategically organized hunting?
15. More organized raw material distribution

moth. These would have provided a rich, if in some contexts slightly unpredictable, food supply for the contemporaneous human groups (Mellars 1985; Mithen 1990).

Following almost a century of debate there now seems to be increasing agreement among both anthropologists and archaeologists that over at least the greater part of Europe the transition from Neanderthal to anatomically modern (or 'Cro-Magnon') populations must reflect a population replacement event, with the anatomically and behaviorally modern populations expanding fairly rapidly from east to west across Europe over the time range from *ca.* 43,000 to 35,000 BP (Stringer & Gamble 1993; Hublin 1990; Mellars 1992; Stringer & McKie 1996; Krings *et al*. 1997; but see Wolpoff *et al*. 1994 and Clark 1997 for conflicting views). Several separate lines of evidence have recently served to reinforce this pattern: The demonstrable presence of essentially anatomically modern human remains in both Israel and parts of Africa by around 100,000 BP — *i.e.,* at least 50–60,000 years before their first appearance in Europe; the extraordinarily abrupt nature of the anatomical interface between the final Neanderthal and early anatomically modern humans — as reflected for example by the anatomical contrasts between the late Neanderthal remains from Saint-Césaire and Le Moustier and the early Cro-Magnon forms from Stetten, Mladec, Cro-Magnon *etc.*; and the rapidly increasing corpus of both nuclear and mitochondrial DNA studies of present-day human populations in different parts of the world which point fairly consistently to a relatively recent origin of the modern human genotype (probably within the last 200,000 years), and its most likely origin at some point in Africa (Aitken *et al*. 1992; Stoneking *et al*. 1992; Harpending *et al*. 1993; Cann *et al*. 1994; Stringer & McKie 1996; Tishkoff *et al*. 1996; Howell 1996; Bräuer *et al*. 1997). Recently, the same case has been greatly strengthened by the recovery of 'ancient' mitochondrial DNA from the original Neanderthal skeleton itself (Krings *et al*. 1997). As we shall see, the archaeological evidence from Europe could be used to argue equally forcibly for an episode of population replacement at this point in the archaeological succession, as opposed to a process of gradual, *in situ,* local evolution from the final Mousterian to the earliest Upper Paleolithic populations (Mellars 1992, 1996a).

The archaeological records spanning the period of the replacement of Neanderthal by anatomically modern populations reflect what I and many other archaeologists (*e.g.,* Pfeiffer 1982; White 1993; Noble & Davidson 1996; Mithen 1996a) would regard as the most radical episode of cultural, technological and general behavioral

change in the entire history of the European continent — at least since the initial colonization of Europe by early *Homo* populations around a million years ago (Table 1).
The term 'Upper Paleolithic Revolution' is now commonly used to describe this transition. As I have discussed in more detail elsewhere, clear and well documented patterns of change at this point can be documented in at least seven or eight separate
features of the archaeological material (Mellars 1973, 1989a, 1989b, 1991, 1996a;
Kozlowski 1990):

1) The appearance of much more widespread 'blade' and 'bladelet' as opposed to
'flake'-based technologies, probably involving the use of new 'punch' techniques of
blade production;

2) The appearance of a wide range of entirely new *forms* of stone tools, some of
which clearly reflect new patterns of technology in other related spheres (such as skin
or bone working, or the construction of new forms of hunting weapons) but others
which seem to reflect an entirely new component of conceptual or visual form and
standardization in the production of stone tools (Mellars 1989b; see below);

3) The effective explosion of bone, antler and ivory technology, involving not
only the appearance of many new techniques for shaping these materials (sawing,
grooving, grinding, polishing, perforating, *etc.*) but a remarkably wide range of new
and tightly standardized tool forms (Figure 1) — again apparently reflecting shifts in
the complexity of several other related areas of technology (Knecht 1993);

4) The appearance of the first reliably documented beads, pendants and other
items of personal decoration (Figure 2) — frequently in large numbers, and manufactured in a range of often difficult materials (*e.g.*, ivory and steatite) by a variety of
manufacturing techniques (White 1989, 1993);

5) The transportation of sea shells and other materials over remarkable distances
of up to 400-600 km — as for example between the Atlantic coasts and Rhone Valley
in France, or between the Adriatic coast and the Danube Valley in Austria (Taborin
1993; Gamble 1986);

6) The appearance of the first unmistakable sound-producing instruments, in the
form of the bird-bone flutes recorded from early Upper Paleolithic levels at sites such
as das Geissenklösterle in Central Europe and Isturitz in the Pyrenees;

7) Most dramatically of all, the sudden appearance of explicitly 'artistic' activity,
in a remarkable variety of forms. From western France we now have simple outlines
of animals engraved on stone blocks, together with engravings of apparently female
sex organs and at least one example of a carved bone phallus (Delluc & Delluc 1978).
From Vogelherd, das Geissenklösterle, Hohlenstein-Stadel and Stratzing in Central
Europe we have a range of carved ivory or stone statuettes of various animal or human
figures (Figure 3), together with one extraordinary composite carving of a male human figure equipped with a lion's head (Figure 4) (Hahn 1972, 1993; Bahn 1994).
And from eastern France dates of 30-32,000 BP have recently been announced for the
series of remarkable drawings of horses, aurochs, rhinos, mammoths and other animals in the cave of Grotte Chauvet in the Ardêche (Chauvet *et al.* 1995; Clottes 1996).
Alongside these more explicitly 'artistic' creations we have a variety of more geometric representations, ranging from regularly spaced lines and crosses engraved on
the surfaces of bone tools to more complex arrangements of dots or liner incisions
which Alexander Marshack (1991) has been tempted to interpret as early forms of nu-
merical notation or even lunar calendars.

The above are the more easily documented archaeological aspects of the so-called
'Upper Paleolithic revolution' in Europe, all clearly documented in the archaeological records in several areas of Europe well before 30,000 BP, and in most cases as

early as 35–40,000 BP (Table 1). The first appearance of all these innovations seems to be closely associated with the earliest appearance of anatomically modern populations, in a way which suggests that the behavioral innovations appeared *with* these new populations (Gambier 1989, 1993). In addition to the various features listed above there are at least strong hints of closely associated changes in several other as-

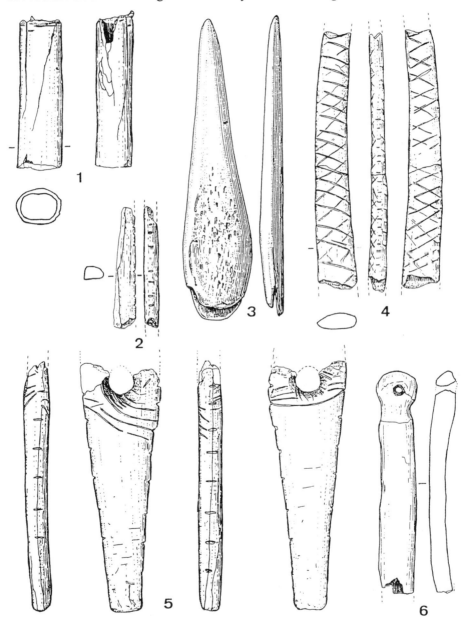

FIGURE 1. Early Upper Paleolithic bone, antler and ivory artifacts from sites in Central Europe, *ca.* 30-40,000 BP.

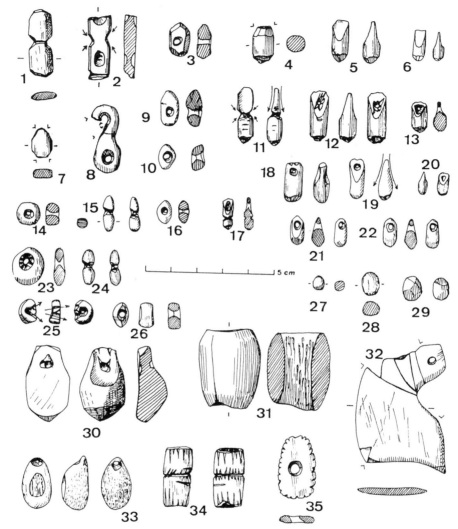

FIGURE 2. Carved ivory beads from Aurignacian levels at the Spy Cave, southern Belgium, *ca* . 30–35,000 BP.

pects of human behavior at broadly the same point in the archaeological sequence — including a sharp increase in the numbers of occupied sites in some of the best documented regions (suggesting a significant increase in human population densities), the appearance of larger and more highly structured occupation sites (in some cases with clear living structures); more large-scale and systematic distribution of raw materials; and in at least certain areas a sharp increase in the degree of specialization in animal exploitation patterns, which at least hints at the emergence of more sharply focused, and probably more 'strategically' organized hunting activities (Mellars 1973, 1989a, 1996a; Stringer & Gamble 1993; Knecht *et al.* 1993). Since the interpretation of some of these features remains more controversial, it may be best for the present discussion to focus on the most easily demonstrated 'facts' of the archaeological record listed in the preceding paragraphs.

The overall impression which emerges therefore is of a fundamental restructuring in almost all of the archaeologically visible aspects of human behavior at this point in the archaeological records of Europe, which appears to correlate closely if not precisely with the anatomical transition from archaic (*i.e.*, Neanderthal) to fully modern populations. If the preceding speculations are correct, this revolution would have extended through almost all spheres of behavior, ranging from several different dimensions of technology, through 'aesthetics,' subsistence patterns, social organization and demography. As several authors have pointed out (*e.g.*, Pfeiffer 1982; White 1989, 1993; Mellars 1989a, 1991; Knight 1991; Donald 1991; Knight *et al.* 1995; Noble & Davidson 1996) the most dramatic single demonstration of this behavioral revolution is in the explicitly 'symbolic' spheres of art, personal ornamentation, ceremonial burial practices, and apparently music. It is this pattern that has led many of us to characterize the so-called Upper Paleolithic revolution as a preeminently *symbolic* revolution — or in John Pfeiffer's (1982) words 'symbolic explosion.' It is the ramifications of this perspective that I will explore below.

The critical question of course is what relevance, if any, does this 'behavioral revolution' or 'symbolic explosion' have for studies of language origins and development in early populations? It is here that one must make a fundamental, but in my

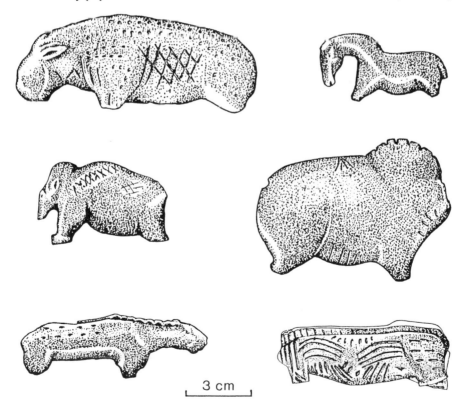

FIGURE 3. Series of animal figures, carved from mammoth ivory, from the early Aurignacian levels of the Vogelherd Cave, southern Germany.

view and that of most other archaeologists and anthropologists, entirely valid assumption — namely, that the extraordinarily complex, highly structured, visually symbol-laden, artistically creative and remarkably 'modern' patterns of culture so explicitly reflected in the archaeological records of Upper Paleolithic populations in

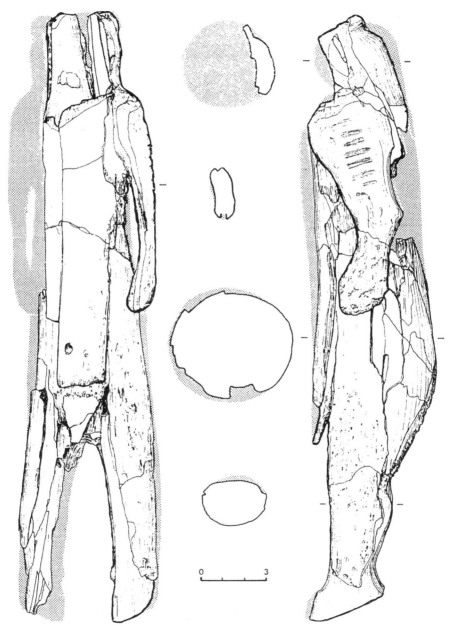

FIGURE 4. Carved mammoth-ivory human figure with a lion's head, from the early Aurignacian levels o f the Hohlenstein-Stadel Cave, southern Germany.

Europe would be inconceivable in the absence of essentially modern, highly structured language. This argument could no doubt be presented in a number of different ways and from a variety of perspectives. It could be argued, for example, that the patterns of technology, subsistence strategies, symbolism, *etc.* documented in many early Upper Paleolithic contexts are at least as complex — and in some cases apparently more complex — than those documented among many of the technologically 'simpler' hunter-gatherer communities of the recent ethnographic past (such as the Tasmanians, or some Bushmen groups), all of which are known to have possessed highly complex, entirely modern language patterns. Other more involved arguments have been constructed relating complex syntax to the creation of complex artistic and representational images (Davidson & Noble 1989, 1993; Noble & Davidson 1996). Leaving aside these more specific arguments, I doubt whether any modern archaeologist, anthropologist or cognitive scientist would seriously dispute that the full panoply of typically Upper Paleolithic culture *must* reflect the presence of essentially modern language patterns among the earliest anatomically modern populations of Europe by at least, say, 35-40,000 years ago (Donald 1991; Bickerton 1990, 1995; Pinker 1994; Gibson 1996; Mithen 1996a, 1996b; Dunbar 1996, *etc.*).

The critical issue in this context therefore hinges on the existence and/or nature of language among the preexisting Neanderthal populations of Europe — and it is on this issue that most of the debate over the past 10–15 years has centered. Some authors (*e.g.*, Binford 1989; Lieberman 1991) have argued that language in any strictly defined sense was probably lacking among the Neanderthal and earlier populations of Europe. Others, including Bickerton (1990, 1995) and myself (1989a, 1996a, 1996b), have taken a less extreme view, while nevertheless accepting that some major shift in the basic complexity or structure of language almost certainly was associated with the Neanderthal to modern human transition. Others of course have taken the view that there is no reason to infer any major contrast between the nature of Neanderthal and modern language (Ragir 1985; Gibson 1996; Mithen 1996b). What follows is an attempt to explore what in my view are the most potentially relevant aspects of the available archaeological evidence to come to grips with this question.

At the outset it seems to me highly unlikely that the Neanderthals possessed no linguistic abilities. As the paper by Peter Marler in the present volume makes clear, many species of primates, and indeed other groups of mammals and birds, have been shown to have relatively complex repertoires of vocal expressions, which seem to convey clear meaning to other members of the groups, even if any form of multiple, sequential symboling or 'syntax' is lacking (see also Parker & Gibson 1990; Pinker 1994; Cheney & Seyfarth 1990, 1996). The Neanderthals of course were separated from our closest primate ancestors by at least five million years of biological and behavioral evolution, had brains around three times the size of any primates, and demonstrably vastly more complicated repertoires of behavior in many different spheres (Stringer & McKie 1996; Mellars 1996a). As Mithen (1996a, 1996b) and others have argued, it seems inconceivable that Neanderthals — and indeed preceding populations of *Homo erectus* and even *Homo habilis* — would not have had systems of vocal communication far more complex than those of any of the living primates.

At the same time however, it would be totally irrational to argue that Neanderthals, simply because they had brains the same size as ours and survived as recently as 30-35,000 years ago, *must* have had linguistic and other cognitive capacities identical to those of modern populations. In brains, as in other spheres, size is not everything, and many earlier studies have demonstrated that brain size alone — or even allometric relationships between brain size and total body size — are notoriously poor indicators of relative cognitive capacities (though the so-called 'neocortex ratio' which relates brain volume to the area of the surrounding neocortex may given a better indication: Aiello & Dunbar 1993; Aiello 1996; Mellars 1996: 368). Clearly, there are many potential functions for large brains quite apart from language (Passingham 1989; Byrne 1996). The crucial point to recognize is that if most of the recent reconstructions of the patterns of human evolution and phylogeny do have any validity, then the line of evolution which led to the European Neanderthals is likely to have been separated from that which led to the evolution of anatomically modern humans over a span of at least 300,000 and probably closer to 500,000 years (Krings *et al.* 1997; also Stringer & McKie 1996; Howell 1996; Bräuer *et al.* 1997) — implying a cumulative evolutionary divergence of these two lineages over a total of at least half a million years. To argue that there can have been no significant change in the neurological complexity of brain structures over this period would plainly be absurd. To argue that the evolution of the brain had effectively come to an end before the evolutionary divergence of the European Neanderthals from the African ancestors of anatomically modern populations would be equally absurd, since this would imply that biological evolutionary processes effectively came to an end at precisely the point when most forms of human interpersonal and intergroup behavioral and social competition are likely to have become most intense (Humphrey 1976; Byrne & Whiten 1988; Dunbar 1996), Clearly, there is no evolutionary or biological justification for assuming that Neanderthals must have had brains identical to ours.

If we turn now to the strictly behavioral and archaeological aspects of the question, I would suggest that there are three features of the available archaeological evidence, in particular, which could be of critical relevance to the nature or structure of Neanderthal language (Table 2; Mellars 1991, 1996a, 1996b):

TABLE 2. Likely behavioral correlates of a 'linguistic revolution.'

1. Symbolic explosion
2. Increased organizational complexity
3. Increased social complexity — especially kinship/descent structures
4. More long-term 'strategic' planning
5. Sharper and more prescribed cultural/ethnic divisions
6. Emergence of complex ideologies, mythologies etc.
7. Increased 'categorical' concepts — *e.g.*, in tool production

The first and most obvious is the virtual lack of convincing evidence for explicitly symbolic thinking or behavior among the Neanderthals. The whole topic of symbolism is of course plagued by semantic and terminological debates and has generated a lively literature (*cf.*, Hodder 1982; Chase 1991; Byers 1994, *etc.*; see Chase 1991 and Mellars 1996a:369 for a discussion of different meanings of symbolism). Without wishing to get too enmeshed in these debates, the most striking feature of the archaeological records of the European Neanderthals is the effective lack of convincing and clearly documented forms of *explicit* symbolism, in the form of clearly representational or even 'geometric' art, obvious items of personal adornment or decoration, or demonstrably 'ritualistic' or 'ceremonial' burial practices (see Chase & Dibble 1987; Gargett 1989; Chase 1991; Mellars 1996a:369–83, 1996b for full documentation of these points). It is true that Neanderthals occasionally used coloring pigments for some as yet unknown purpose, sporadically collected unusual or intriguing fossil shells (though with no evidence for their use for personal ornaments) and certainly buried human corpses in simple, unadorned graves in their cave or rock-shelter living sites. But none of this in my view necessarily implies anything clearly symbolic in the activities represented (Mellars 1996a, 1996b; Chase & Dibble 1987; Chase 1991), and certainly pales into virtual insignificance when set beside the dramatic explosion of decorative, ornamental, artistic and other explicitly symbolic activities and arti-facts recorded from scores of early Upper Paleolithic sites across the length and breadth of Europe (White 1989, 1993).

The linkages between visual symbolism and language can no doubt be argued in many ways (see for example Davidson and Noble 1989, 1993; Donald 1991; Knight 1991; Mithen 1996a; Noble & Davidson 1996, *etc.*). No one would question however that language is, *par excellence*, a highly symbolic activity and, as Merlin Donald (1991) and others have argued, one might reasonably predict that any sudden intro-duction of highly elaborate and symbolic forms of linguistic communication would be accompanied by a corresponding increase in the range and complexity of visual and ceremonial symbolism. In other words it would not be surprising if the 'symbolic explosion' in archaeological terms coincided with a 'linguistic explosion' in cogni-tive and communication terms.

The second, more direct correlation I have proposed between the archaeological record and language lies in the essentially new element of clearly 'imposed form' and 'visual standardization' in artifact production which I believe represents one of the most striking general features of the archaeological transition from the Middle to the Upper Paleolithic (Mellars 1989b, 1991, 1996b). The essence of this idea is that while Middle Paleolithic craftsmen were unquestionably expert flint knappers and clearly invested a good deal of time and effort into producing *functionally* efficient and varied tool forms, they seem with a few rare and debatable exceptions (notably bi-faces: see Mellars 1996a:135–6; Gowlett 1996) to have shown surprisingly little con-cern with the overall visual appearance of the tools. As a result, Middle Paleolithic stone tools seem to grade almost imperceptibly — and to an archaeological taxono-mist extremely irritatingly — between 'convergent sidescapers' and 'points,' be-tween 'bifacial racloirs' and 'handaxes,' between 'notches' and 'denticulates,' and so on (see also Chase & Dibble 1987; Dibble 1989). Anyone who has tried to teach Mousterian typology to students will be acutely aware of the problem of attempting to neatly categorize or classify Middle Paleolithic stone tools into clearly separated 'types' or discrete morphological forms.

By contrast, Upper Paleolithic stone tool types not only show a vastly greater range of morphological diversity than Middle Paleolithic tools (diversity which, as discussed below, changes rapidly over both space and time) but also a much more ob-vious degree of repetition and standardization in the visual *appearance* of the tools. In most cases this was achieved by flaking away a good deal of the original blade or flake blank until some relatively standardized and normally highly distinctive visual form was *imposed* on the tool. As I have commented elsewhere (Mellars 1991:66), it is as though Upper Paleolithic flint workers were saying "this is an end-scraper: I use it as an end-scraper, I call it an end-scraper and it must therefore *look* like an end-scraper," whereas Middle Paleolithic groups seem to have been content with the maxim "who cares what this tool looks like as long as it functions adequately for the job in hand." This same element of visually imposed form and morphological stan-dardization is arguably even more conspicuous in many of the major types of Upper Paleolithic bone, antler and ivory tools, as well as in various forms of personal orna-ments, artistic motifs and even in the clearly 'structured' form of many Upper Paleo-lithic occupation sites (Mellars 1991, 1996a:381–3)

To cut a potentially rather complicated argument short (Mellars 1991; 1996a: 133-6, 381-3), my contention is that this kind of greatly increased emphasis on the visual morphology and appearance of tools, and the sharply defined separation of the different tool forms into relatively standardized and clearly separated visual categories, is probably exactly what one would anticipate if Upper Paleolithic groups had a much more complex and highly structured *vocabulary* for the different artefacts forms. The contention here is simply that words and names are essentially devices for breaking up what are often continuously varying shapes or concepts into a range of *discrete, categorical* entities — much as we divide the continuously varying colors of the rainbow into "red," "orange," "yellow," "green," *etc.* In other words one can argue that where a name exists, there must presumably be some distinctive visual or mental image (or 'mental template') to go with it. If I use the word 'spoon' for example, this immediately evokes not only the notion of something which can be used to eat soup, but a distinctive visual image, with a rounded bowl, elongated, splayed handle, curved profile, *etc.* In the present context, all of this would make sense if, for example, Neanderthal groups had just one or two names for stone tools, whereas Upper Paleolithic groups had perhaps ten or twenty. At the very least it could be used to argue for a greatly increased linguistic vocabulary over the period of the Middle-Upper Paleolithic transition. When we add to this the even greater degree of complexity of bone, antler and ivory tools in the Upper Paleolithic, various forms of personal ornaments and decorative items, artistic representations, *etc.*, the scale of contrast purely at the level of the complexity of vocabularies in the two periods could be fairly dramatic.

One final and much more general aspect of the archaeological records of the Middle and Upper Paleolithic which has been stressed by Binford, Whallon and others as potentially highly relevant to the nature and complexity of language is the overall degree of complexity reflected in different spheres of the behavior, organization and strategic 'planning' of Neanderthal and anatomically modern groups. As Whallon (1989) in particular has argued, the emergence of highly structured language, with complex syntax, past and future tenses, subordinate clauses, subjunctives, *etc.* would almost inevitably have had a profound on the capacity for human groups to organize and structure all aspects of their activities, ranging from the planning and coordination of hunting expeditions, through the construction of elaborate myths, belief systems and ideologies, to the patterns of social roles and relationships between individuals in the groups — including for example the recognition of complex systems of kinship and descent (see also Donald 1991; Knight 1991; Rodseth *et al.* 1991; Bickerton 1990; Dunbar 1996; Mellars 1996c; *etc.*). Binford (1989) has emphasized the role of language in what he refers to as 'long-range planning' — the capacity to conceptualize and organize activities (including more long-term plans for tool production and 'curation,' or the long term use of occupation sites) over periods of more than a few hours or a few days. In this context the evidence for apparently more highly specialized and strategically organized hunting patterns in the Upper Paleolithic, more highly organized systems for the long-range procurement and distribution of raw materials, and larger and more structured occupation sites could all be highly significant (Mellars 1996a). Indeed, Whallon (1989) and Soffer (1994) have argued that the appearance of fully complex language could have been the critical factor which allowed the first permanent occupation of some of the more extreme periglacial environments in central and eastern Europe which seem to have been largely if not entirely avoided by Neanderthal groups.

There is one further aspect of the archaeological transition from the Middle to the Upper Paleolithic which is potentially highly relevant to the emergence of language but which to my knowledge has never been specifically discussed in these terms. This is the very much sharper degree of both chronological and spatial variations in technology documented throughout the European Upper Paleolithic in comparison to that in the Middle Paleolithic. The archaeological reality of this contrast has of course been commented on frequently in the earlier literature (*e.g.*, Isaac 1972; Gamble 1986; Sackett 1988; Klein 1989) and is to some extent a commonplace of the Paleolithic record. This is emphatically not to suggest that *no* significant variations can be detected in Middle Paleolithic/Neanderthal technologies in Europe — both chronological and spatial — as I myself have argued at length (*e.g.*, 1969, 1992, 1996a). The point is simply that variations of this kind are not only reflected in far more striking and idiosyncratic terms in the Upper Paleolithic — that is by a welter of visually striking and distinctive 'type-fossil' forms in both stone tools and bone/antler implements (Mellars 1989b) — but also that the individual chronological and spatial units of variation change over a much more rapid time-scale in the Upper than in the Middle Paleolithic. In the classic Upper Paleolithic sequence of western Europe for example we can now recognize at least 15–20 discrete technological stages over a total period of *ca.* 30,000 years, most of them defined by effectively unique type-fossil forms which change at intervals of every few thousand years (de Sonneville-Bordes 1961; Bordes 1984; Sackett 1988). In at least many stages of the Upper Paleolithic sequence similar complexity can be documented in the geographical distribution of different industries. Thus the various stages of the Solutrian and most of the classic variants of the Magdalenian are restricted to western Europe (Smith 1966; Bosinski 1990); the Noaillian is confined essentially to southern France and northern Italy (David 1985); a variety of distinctive regional variants can be recognized in different areas of the west European Solutrian (Smith 1964, 1966); and a similar range of regional variants in the central and eastern European Gravettian (Otte 1981; Kozlowski & Kozlowski 1979). Whatever degree of chronological and regional variation can be recognized within the technology of Neanderthal communities in Europe is exceeded by a least an order of magnitude in the technologies of Upper Paleolithic groups.

The generally held view among Paleolithic specialists is that this greatly increased degree of technological and typological variation in the European Upper Paleolithic is in some way reflecting both a much more sharply defined pattern of ethnic divisions among Upper Paleolithic groups — apparent in a strong component of 'style' in the associated artefacts — and the emergence of strong cultural, social and ethnic *traditions*, which led to the clearly defined inheritance of these technological and stylistic features from one generation to the next (Isaac 1972; Jochim 1983; Gamble 1986; Sackett 1988; Mellars 1989b; Shennan 1996). In the context of the present discussion I would suggest that both of these features are precisely what one would predict if complex, highly structured language emerged for the first time in the Upper Paleolithic. There are three main strands to the argument. The first is that [as Donald (1991) and others have argued] language is probably essential to the effective transmission of tightly defined rules of complex social and cultural behavior from one generation to the next, and is therefore at least a strong catalyst to the emergence of sharply defined cultural traditions, if not an essential prerequisite. The second is that language is arguably the most important single factor in unifying the culture and behavior of specific social groups, and therefore maintaining this kind of ethnicity in the material record (Wiessner 1983, 1984). The third, of course, is that linguistic differences, once established, become by far the most powerful and effective means of reinforcing and maintaining social *divisions* between distinct ethnic groups — as for example all the literature on documented tribal divisions in recent hunter-gatherer communities clearly reveals (*e.g.*, Peterson 1976). In short, if there was indeed a 'revolution' in the complexity and structure of language over the period of the Neanderthal to modern human transition in Europe, one should perhaps expect to see as an automatic concomitant of this a much sharper degree of divergence and rapid change in the associated material cultures. Moreover it would not be unreasonable to suggest that at least some of the geographical and chronological divergences in material culture documented throughout the Upper Paleolithic sequence may be reflecting fairly directly corresponding divergences in language patterns (see Renfrew, this volume).

The inference I am drawing from all the preceding lines of evidence is that whereas Neanderthal communities in Europe almost certainly had some form of language, and while this is likely to have been far more complex and highly structured than that of any of the present-day primates, Neanderthal language patterns most probably were still radically simpler in certain fundamental respects than those of the succeeding Upper Paleolithic populations. I have suggested that two of the critical differences may have been a much more limited vocabulary or lexicon, and probably a much more rudimentary pattern of grammar and syntax, which severely restricted the range and complexity of verbal communications.   Lieberman, of course, has drawn essentially the same conclusion based on certain anatomical details of the Neanderthal skull and associated larynx (Lieberman 1989, 1990), though these interpretations have been disputed by others (*e.g.*, Ahrensburg 1989). The implication in other words is that the Neanderthal — sand probably earlier populations of *Homo erectus* and possibly *Homo habilis* — possessed some form of 'protolanguage.' One of the main challenges at present is to construct explicit models of exactly what form these evolutionary 'protolanguages' might have taken, since I believe it is only by constructing explicit models for alternative patterns of language development that we will be able to test these potential models effectively against the archaeological evidence. At present I am aware of only one really explicit attempt of this kind. This is embodied in Derek Bickerton's (1990, 1995) suggestion that the development of language in the course of human evolution is likely to have paralleled that of the ontogenetic development of language in young children — *i.e.*, that at least in language development 'phylogeny may recapitulate ontogeny.' On this basis he has outlined a pattern of 'protolanguage' which he suggests may have resembled that of 1½–2 year old children in containing only very simple, 'here-and-now' sentences, lacking any complex syntax, and virtually lacking the ability to refer to objects or events 'displaced' in time or space from the present. He argues from both the patterns of language development in young children and from similar transformations between pidgin and creole languages in recent language-contact situations that the transition from 'proto' to 'full' language is likely by its nature to have been relatively abrupt, with few if any potentially intermediate stages (Bickerton 1990:164–74). Of course, all of this is controversial. If true it would argue for a remarkably abrupt, essentially quantum-leap event in the evolutionary development of language, presumably involving some fairly dramatic genetic mutation in the course of human evolution. Nevertheless the hypothetical pattern which Bickerton has suggested for the nature of his 'protolanguage' could well correspond fairly closely with some of the speculations outlined above for the language of the European Neanderthals.

As a final point we should perhaps turn to Mithen's recent suggestion that the essence of the contrast between Neanderthal as opposed to fully modern cognition lay in the transition from what he refers to as 'modular' or 'domain-specific' to 'generalized' intelligence (Mithen 1996a, 1996b). The central argument, drawing on the work of Tooby & Cosmides (1992) and others, is that separate, highly specialized components of cognition — including language — emerged fairly gradually in the course of human evolution, in response to specific selective pressures acting on equally specific areas of behavior — tool manufacture, food acquisition, social relationships, communication, *etc*. Only later, at the time of the classic Middle-to-Upper Paleolithic transition, did these different domains of intelligence finally coalesce to generate fully modern, much more fluid and flexible forms of intelligence. These are all plausible suggestions, which would fit well with many aspects of the archaeological records of the Neanderthals as well as with much of the recent thinking by evolutionary psychologists on the evolutionary development of intelligence. With regard to Mithen's speculations on the origins of language, however, three specific questions spring to mind:

1) How plausible is it that the kind of relatively sudden integration of different, previously separate spheres of intelligence into a single 'generalized' intelligence could occur *without* some equally direct and fairly dramatic impact on the structure and complexity of language?

2) If this kind of direct impact on language should be seen as an almost inevitable concomitant of the processes he is proposing, in what sense is he challenging the notion that the 'Upper Paleolithic revolution' was also in some sense a linguistic revolution?

3) Thirdly, could we not in fact reverse the direction of the cause and effect relationships that Mithen has in mind and suggest that it could well have been the evolutionary emergence of fully modern linguistic structures which *allowed* the integration of the previously separated modular cognitive domains in the human mind?

We could pose a broadly similar set of questions in relation to Bickerton's recent arguments (outlined above) that the evolutionary emergence of fully modern language must, by its nature, have been a relatively sudden, 'catastrophic' event, rather than a slow and gradual shift in increasing linguistic complexity. For all the reasons which have been spelled out by Bickerton himself (1990, 1995), Whallon (1989), Donald (1991), Knight (1991), Pinker (1994) and others, any sudden transformation in the complexity and structure of language would almost inevitably have fairly radical consequences for virtually all aspects of human organization and behavior — ranging from technology, through subsistence strategies, social structures, communication patterns, ideological and mythological beliefs etc. The critical question in this case is exactly where, in the archaeological records of the European Paleolithic, might one identify this kind of behavioral watershed, if *not* over the period of the Middle-Upper Paleolithic transition (Mellars 1996a:391)?

Discussion

In the preceding sections I have argued that in the archaeological records of Europe there was probably a radical shift in the overall complexity and structure of language associated closely with the archaeological transition from the Middle to the Upper Paleolithic, and with the associated transition from Neanderthal to fully anatomically modern humans. I have tried to identify what may be the most relevant aspects of human behavior for inferring the emergence of more complex and highly structured language, and discussed how these might be reflected in the surviving archaeological records (Table 2). Following the policy of working from the known to the unknown, this has hopefully put at least some of the basic elements of the linguistic jigsaw into place.

Exactly what relevance all of this has for the more distant evolutionary origins of language is of course an entirely separate question. As discussed in the introduction, it is now clear that the transition from Neanderthal to fully modern populations in Europe almost certainly represents a major population replacement event, with the biologically and behaviorally modern populations dispersing fairly rapidly across Europe from some external source. Although debates continue, several different strands of the evidence point increasingly to Africa as the most likely point of origin of the genetically modern populations (Harpending et al. 1993; Cann *et al.* 1994; Tishkoff *et al.* 1996; Stringer & McKie 1996; Howell 1996). The evidence suggests that some of these populations may initially have spread from Africa as early as 100,000 years ago — although the possibility of more than one dispersal event has sometimes been discussed (Lahr & Foley 1994; Foley & Lahr 1997). But in any event, the populations which spread across Europe around 40,000 years ago are likely to have had their biological and behavioral origins well beyond the bounds of Europe, and well before the date of 40,000 BP.

The obvious question therefore arises as to how far we can identify evidence for the initial emergence of some of the more culturally and cognitively advanced patterns of behavior — including language — in areas beyond Europe, and especially within the hypothetical homeland of the anatomically modern populations in, or close to, Africa. Here we immediately encounter the problem that the intensity of archaeological research on African sites within the relevant time range (*i.e.*, between say 50,000 and 100,000 BP) has been much less than in Europe, so that the degree of detail and resolution of the archaeological records is much less. Nevertheless there are at least three features of the available archaeological evidence from Africa and closely adjacent areas which could be held to provide at least some strong hints that the emergence of more complex, broadly 'Upper Paleolithic'-like behavioral patterns — and most probably language — may be significantly earlier in these areas than in Europe:

1) The first is that remarkable archaeological phenomenon known as the 'Howieson's Poort' industries, now documented from a range of sites in southern Africa to the south of the Zambezi (Deacon 1989; Clark 1992). Precise dating of these industries is still slightly controversial, but most estimates place them at around 50-75,000 BP, certainly long before the emergence of typically Upper Paleolithic technologies in Europe (Grun *et al.* 1990). The remarkable feature of the Howieson's Poort industries is their strikingly Upper Paleolithic-like appearance (Figure 5), including not only typical blade technology but also classic forms of end scrapers and burins, and a range of carefully shaped, semi-microlithic trapeze and crescent shaped forms which not only reflect a high degree of standardization and visually "imposed form," but which almost certainly indicate the presence of complex, multicomponent hunting projectiles at this early date (Deacon 1989). Apparently associated with this industry at the site of Klasies River Mouth was at least one specimen of a carefully shaped bone point and two specimens of regularly notched bones, which again would be much more at home in an Upper than a Middle Paleolithic context in Europe (Singer & Wymer 1982). Overall the African Howiesons Poort industries could be seen as evidence of the emergence of at least the major technological components of typically Upper Paleolithic culture at least 10–20,000 years earlier in southern Africa than in either Europe or Asia (Mellars 1989a:367-9).

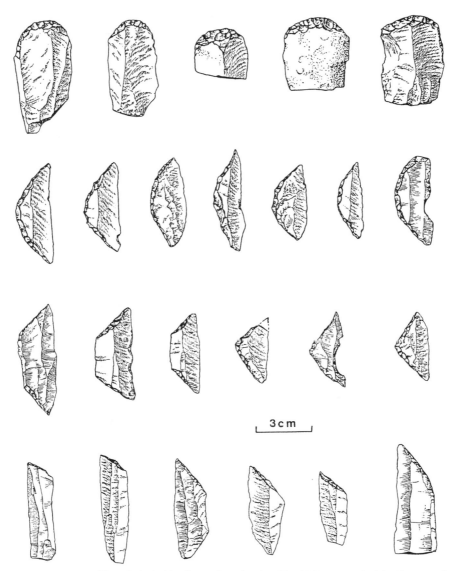

FIGURE 5. Stone artifacts from the Howiesons Poort levels (50?–75,000 BP) at Klasie's River Mouth, South Africa, showing a range of microlithic crescents, triangles, end scrapers and other characteristically Upper Paleolithic forms.

2) The second feature is the striking abundance of coloring pigments recorded at many African sites within the general time range of 40–100,000 BP. As Knight, Power, and Watts (1995) have recently documented, the evidence comes in the form not only of large quantities of red and yellow ocher recorded from many Middle Stone Age sites, but also the presence of clear 'pencils' or 'crayons' of ocher, and a number of stone slabs heavily smeared with ocher which appear to represent coloring palettes. While fragments of ocher are by no means unknown in Neanderthal contexts in Europe (Mellars 1996a), the evidence does seem to suggest a more intensive use of

coloring materials in Africa than in contemporaneous European contexts. It is tempting of course to suggest that this might reflect a much more enterprising use of pigments in these early African sites than among the European Neanderthals, conceivably involving the earliest stages of symbolic or 'artistic' representation. Unfortunately, any direct evidence of how the coloring materials were employed is at present lacking.

3) Thirdly, moving just beyond the bounds of Africa, there are the remarkable burials associated with the essentially anatomically modern skeletons from the two sites of Skhul and Qafzeh in Israel, both now securely dated to around 90–100,000 BP (Bar-Yosef 1992, 1994, 1996). The unique feature of these burials, in contrast to those of the European Neanderthals, is the presence in each case of unmistakable grave offerings (Figure 6), in the form of a complete boar's jaw reputedly 'clasped in the arms' of one of the skeletons at Skhul, and a large fallow deer antler placed immediately on top of one of the burials at Qafzeh (Defleur 1993; Vandermeersch 1970,

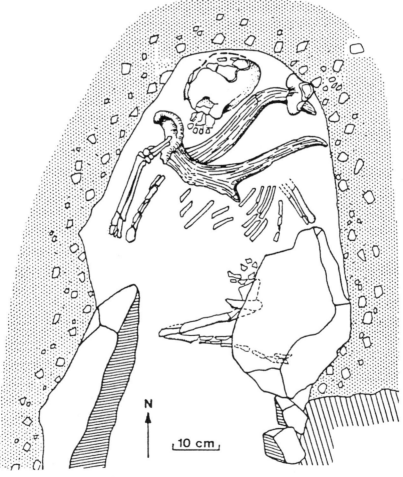

FIGURE 6. Burial of an anatomically modern skeleton accompanied by a large fallow deer antler, from the site of Qafzeh, Israel, dated to *ca*. 100,000 BP.

1976). Once again, the evidence could be seen as a reflection of a significantly more symbolic or 'ceremonial' approach to burial ritual in these Israeli sites at this early date than in anything at present recorded at the same time in Europe. These discoveries of course are located only immediately beyond the limits of northeast Africa and are generally seen as evidence for a brief, temporary incursion of anatomically modern human populations into southwest Asia around the beginning of the last glacial period (Bar-Yosef 1992).

The evidence cited above remains limited, but is nevertheless consistent with the hypothesis of a significantly earlier emergence of various forms of explicitly symbolic behavior in areas either in or closely adjacent to Africa than in other parts of the world. In terms of possible criteria for the emergence of increasingly complex and highly structured language discussed earlier, this could be fully consistent with current models for an essentially African origin for the early evolution of genetically modern populations, implied by recent studies of both the anatomical and genetic evidence (Harpending *et al.* 1993; Stringer & McKie 1996; Howell 1996). In language, as in other aspects of our genetic and biological make-up, the evolutionary source of 'modern' human populations could very well be African.

Cognitive Capacity and Cultural Performance:
The 'Sapient Paradox'

There is one final point which should be raised here, since this seems to have emerged as a source of considerable confusion in some of the recent literature, and indeed surfaced in the discussions at the present conference. This is the need to make a clear and fundamental distinction between the notions of *cognitive potential* and *behavioral performance* in discussions of the emergence of fully modern behavior and associated language in human evolution (*cf.* Mellars 1991:70; Renfrew 1996). There is an obvious and unfortunate asymmetry in the nature of the evidence here. While it is obviously (and by definition) true that no individual or human group can perform *above* the level of their biological and cognitive capacities, it is equally self-evident that people can, and very frequently do, perform *below* their full capacities. In other words, while some patterns of behavior in the archaeological record can easily be held up as concrete proof that the necessary cognitive capacities for that form of behavior existed in the populations in question, the *absence* of these patterns of behavior need not imply that the essential capacities for the behavior were lacking. The absence of particular patterns of behavior or cultural expression in particular societies could be due to a whole range of factors: the lack of a specific need or stimulus for that behavior in particular economic, social or environmental contexts; the lack of adequate raw materials to support particular technological processes; or indeed the simple fact (or historical accident) that particular aspects of behavior or technology had not yet been developed or 'invented' by the societies in question. Clearly, the lack of advanced metal technology or knowledge of mathematics in recent hunter-gatherer communities in no way reflects any lack of the basic cognitive capacities for these behaviors in the societies in question, still less any cognitive inferiority to modern industrialized societies. Similarly the failure to use computers in ancient Rome did not reflect any lack of mental capacities to develop or operate computers. In all these cases technology and other aspects of behavior for various reasons either had not 'caught up' with the full mental capacities of the societies in question, or was simply not necessary, appropriate, or (in some cases) possible in the specific social, economic and environmental contexts of the societies involved.

These points are all very obvious but may help to resolve some of the recurrent confusions in recent discussions of the emergence of fully modern behavior. A full discussion of all the relevant issues would no doubt require a separate paper. But recognition of these points could well explain, for example, while the early anatomically modern populations represented at Skhul and Qafzeh in Israel (at around 100,000 BP) were still employing technologies that we describe in archaeological terms as essentially 'Middle' as opposed to 'Upper' Paleolithic (Bar-Yosef 1992, 1994). Lithic technology of course represents only a minute fraction of the total behavioral and adaptive repertoire of any human group, and it could well be that in many other spheres the behavior and organization of the Skhul/Qafzeh populations was essentially 'modern' (*cf.* Lieberman & Shea 1994). In this context, as noted above, the presence of what appear to be demonstrably ceremonial burial rites at both sites could well be highly significant (Figure 6). Similar factors almost certainly explain why some of the most impressive aspects of complex bone, antler and ivory technology, personal ornamentation, and various forms of art are far more conspicuous in the archaeological records of the European Upper Paleolithic than in those of the Middle East, Africa and parts of Asia. As several authors have pointed out (*e.g.*, Oswalt 1976; Price & Brown 1985), a variety of different environmental and related economic and demographic factors tend to favor more complex patterns of social organization and associated material culture among societies occupying highly stressed and economically unpredictable arctic or periglacial environments than in those occupying less-demanding temperate or tropical environments. And the absence of highly developed blade technology in many contexts simply reflects the heavy requirements which blade technology imposes on both the quality and nodule-size of available raw material supplies. Even in some classic European Upper Paleolithic contexts blade technology may be virtually lacking in certain situations where good raw materials are not locally available — as for example at El Castillo and some other sites in northern Spain or in many of the Upper Paleolithic industries of the west Italian coast (Strauss & Heller 1988; Cabrera Valdés 1984; Mussi 1992). How far similar considerations may explain the lack of classic blade-based technologies over large areas of eastern and southeast Asia and Australasia is an interesting point for speculation (Mellars 1989a:377; Schick & Toth 1993; Lourandos 1996) — especially if we remember that any technology has to adapt to the *overall* levels of environmental constraints in any region, and not just to small, isolated 'windows' of environmental opportunity.

The purpose of this discussion is to emphasize that the absence of highly developed, classically Upper Paleolithic-like technologies in many contexts need not in any sense imply the lack of fully modern cognitive capacities, nor the absence of fully developed language. The asymmetry of the evidence for *cognitive potential* as opposed to *behavioral performance* must be kept clearly in mind here. In my view the emergence of what appear to be typically Upper Paleolithic technologies at Klasie's River Mouth and other early sites in southern Africa may well provide strong evidence for the emergence of fully modern cognitive and language capacities in this area at a substantially earlier date than in Europe. The *absence* of the full panoply of Upper Paleolithic technologies in certain other contexts demonstrably associated with anatomically modern humans on the other hand need not imply a lack of these capacities, for all the reasons outlined above. The fact remains that the most dramatic event in the history of European populations is reflected in the classic 'Upper Paleolithic revolution,' which occurred closely if not precisely in association with the appearance of the first anatomically modern populations. I would suggest that in this case the archaeological evidence almost certainly is reflecting some form of cognitive and linguistic revolution, and that this revolution was introduced into Europe by the arrival of new populations, most probably from an ultimately African source.

Literature Cited

Aiello, L.C. 1996. Hominine preadaptations for language and cognition. Pages 89–99 *in* P. Mellars & K. Gibson, eds., *Modeling the Early Human Mind.* McDonald Institute for Archaeological Research, Cambridge, U.K.

Aiello, L.C., & R. Dunbar. 1993. Neocortex size, group size and the evolution of language. *Curr. Anthropol.* 34:184–193.

Aitken, M., C. Stringer, & P. Mellars, eds. 1992. *The Origin of Modern Humans and the Impact of Chronometric Dating.* Royal Society (Philosophical Transactions of the Royal Society, series B, 337, no. 1280), London, U.K.

Aitchison, J. 1996. *The Seeds of Speech: Language Origin and Evolution.* Cambridge University Press, Cambridge, U.K.

Arensburg, B. 1989. New skeletal evidence concerning the anatomy of Middle Paleolithic populations in the Middle East:The Kebara skeleton. Pages 165–171 *in* P. Mellars & C. Stringer, eds., *The Human Revolution: Behavioral and Biological Perspectives on the Origins of Modern Humans.* Princeton University Press, Princeton.

Bahn, P.G. 1994. New advances in the field of ice age art. Pages 121–132 *in* M.H. Nitecki & D.V. Nitecki, eds., *Origins of Anatomically Modern Humans.* Plenum Press, New York.

Bar-Yosef, O. 1992. The role of western Asia in modern human origins. Pages 193–200 *in* M.J. Aitken, C.B. Stringer, & P.A. Mellars, eds., *The Origin of Modern Humans and the Impact of Chronometric Dating.* Royal Society (Philosophical Transactions of the Royal Society, series B, 337, no. 1280), London, U.K.

————. 1994. The contribution of southwest Asia to the study of the origins of modern humans. Pages 23–66 *in* M.T. Nitecki & D. V. Nitecki, eds, *Origins of Anatomically Modern Humans.* Plenum Press, New York.

————. 1996. Modern humans, Neanderthals and the Middle/Upper Paleolithic transition in western Asia. Pages 175–190 *in* M. Piperno, ed.,*The Lower and Middle Paleolithic: Colloquia.* XIII International Congress of Prehistoric and Protohistoric Sciences, Forli, Italy.

Bard, E., B. Hamelin, R.G. Fairbanks, & A. Zindler. 1990. Calibration of the ^{14}C timescale over the past 30,000 years using mass spectrometric U-Th ages from Barbados corals. *Nature* 354:405–410.

Bickerton, D. 1990. *Language and Species.* University of Chicago Press, Chicago.

————. 1995. *Language and Human Behavior.* University of Washington Press, Seattle.

Binford, L.R. 1989. Isolating the transition to cultural adaptations: An organizational approach. Pages 18–41 *in* E. Trinkaus, ed., *The Emergence of Modern Humans: Biocultural Adaptations in the Later Pleistocene.* Cambridge University Press, Cambridge, U.K.

Bordes, F. 1984. *Leçons sur le Paléolithique: vol. 2: Le Paléolithique en Europe.* Centre National de la Recherche Scientifique (Institut du Quaternaire, Université de Bordeaux I, Cahiers du Quaternaire no. 7), Paris, France.

Bosinski, G. 1990. *Homo Sapiens.* Editions France, Paris, France.

Bräuer, G., Y. Yokoyama, C. Falgueres, & E. Mbua. 1997. Modern human origins backdated. *Nature* 386:337.

Byers, A.M. 1994. Symboling and the Middle-Upper Paleolithic transition: a theoretical and methodological critique. *Curr. Anthropol.* 35:369–399.

Byrne, R.W. 1996. Relating brain size to intelligence in primates. Pages 49–56 *in* P. Mellars & K. Gibson, eds, *Modeling the Early Human Mind*. McDonald Institute for Archaeological Research, Cambridge, U.K.

Byrne, R.W. & A. Whiten. 1988. *Machiavellian Intelligence: Social Expertise and the Evolution of Intellect in Monkeys, Apes and Humans*. Oxford University Press, Oxford, U.K.

———. 1992. Cognitive evolution in primates: evidence from tactical deception. *Man* 27:609–627.

Cabrera Valdés, V. 1984. *El Yacimento de la Cueva de "El Castillo" (Puente Viesgo, Santander)*. Bibliotheca Praehistorica Hispana, vol. XXII, Madrid, Spain.

Cann, R.L., O. Rickards, & J. Koji Lum. 1994. Mitochondrial DNA and human evolution: Our one lucky mother. Pages 135–148 *in* M.H. Nitecki & D.V. Nitecki, eds., *Origins of Anatomically Modern Humans*. Plenum Press, New York.

Chase, P.G. 1991. Symbols and Paleolithic artifacts: style, standardization, and the imposition of arbitrary form. *Jour. Anthropol. Archeol.* 10:193–214.

Chase, P.G. & H.L. Dibble. 1987. Middle Paleolithic symbolism: A review of current evidence and interpretations. *Jour. Anthropol. Archeol.* 6:263–296.

Chauvet, J.-M., E.B. Deschamps, & C. Hillaire. 1995. *La Grotte Chauvet*. Seuil, Paris, France.

Cheney, D.L. & R.M. Seyfarth. 1990. *How Monkeys see the World: Inside the Mind of Another Species*. University of Chicago Press, Chicago.

———. 1996. Function and intention in the calls of non-human primates. Pages 59–76 *in* W.G. Runciman, J. Maynard Smith, & R.I. Dunbar, eds., *The Evolution of Social Behaviour Patterns in Primates and Man*. Oxford University Press (Proceedings of the British Academy, vol. 88), Oxford, U.K.

Clark, J.D. 1992. African and Asian perspectives on the origins of modern humans. Pages 201–216 *in* M. Aitken, C.B. Stringer, & P.A. Mellars, eds, *The Origin of Modern Humans and the Impact of Chronometric Dating*. Royal Society (Philosophical Transactions of the Royal Society, series B, 337, no. 1280), London, U.K.

Clark, G.A. 1997. The Middle-Upper Paleolithic transition in Europe: an American perspective. *Norweg. Archaeol. Rev.* 30:25–53.

Clottes, J. 1996. Recent studies on Paleolithic art. *Cambr. Archaeol. Jour.* 6:179–189.

David, N.C. 1985. *Excavation of the Abri Pataud, Les Eyzies (Dordogne) France: The Noaillian (level 4) Assemblage and the Noaillian Culture in Western Europe*. Peabody Museum, Harvard University, Cambridge.

Davidson, I. & W. Noble. 1989. The archaeology of perception: Traces of depiction and language. *Curr. Anthropol.* 30:125–155.

———. 1993. Tools and language in human evolution. Pages 363–387 *in* K.R. Gibson & T. Ingold, eds., *Tools, Language and Cognition in Human Evolution*. Cambridge University Press, Cambridge, U.K.

Deacon, H. 1989. Late Pleistocene palaeoecology and archaeology in the southern Cape, South Africa. Pages 547–564 *in* P. Mellars & C. Stringer, eds, *The Human Revolution: Behavioral and Biological Perspectives on the Origins of Modern Humans*. Princeton University Press, Princeton.

Defleur, A. 1993. *Les Sépultures Moustériennes*. CNRS, Paris, France.

Delluc, B. & G. Delluc. 1978. Les manifestations graphiques aurignaciennes sur support rocheux des environs des Eyzies (Dordogne) *Gallia-Préhistoire* 21:213–438.

Dibble, H.L. 1989. The implications of stone tool types for the presence of language in the Lower and Middle Paleolithic. Pages 415–432 *in* P. Mellars & C. Stringer, eds., *The Hu-*

man Revolution: Behavioral and Biological Perspectives on the Origins of Modern Humans. Princeton University Press, Princeton.

Donald, M. 1991. *Origins of the Modern Mind: Three Stages in the Evolution of Culture and Cognition*. Harvard University Press, Cambridge.

Dunbar, R. 1996. *Grooming, Gossip and the Evolution of Language*. Faber & Faber, London, U.K.

Farizy, C., ed. 1990. *Paléolithique Moyen Récent et Paléolithique Supérieur Ancien en Europe*. Mémoires du Musée de Préhistoire d'Ile de France, Nemours, France.

Foley, R. & M.M. Lahr. 1997. Mode 3 technologies and the evolution of modern humans. *Cambr. Archaeol. Jour.* 7:3–36.

Gambier, D. 1989. Fossil hominids from the early Upper Paleolithic (Aurignacian) of France. Pages 194–211 *in* P. Mellars & C. Stringer, eds., *The Human Revolution: Behavioral and Biological Perspectives on the Origins of Modern Humans*. Princeton University Press, Princeton.

————. 1993. Les hommes modernes du debut du Paléolithique supérieur en France: bilan des données anthropologiques et perspectives. Pages 409–430 *in* V. Cabrera Valdés, ed., *El Origen del Hombre Moderno en el Suroeste de Europa*. Madrid: Universidad Nacional de Educacion a Distancia, Spain.

Gamble, C. 1986. *The Paleolithic Settlement of Europe*. Cambridge University Press, Cambridge, U.K.

Gargett, R.H. 1989. Grave shortcomings: The evidence for Neanderthal burial. *Curr. Anthropol.* 30:157–90.

Gibson, K. R. 1996. The biocultural human brain, seasonal migrations, and the emergence of the Upper Paleolithic. Pages 33–46 *in* P. Mellars & K. Gibson, eds., *Modeling the Early Human Mind*. McDonald Institute for Archaeological Research, Cambridge, U.K.

Gibson, K.R. & T. Ingold. 1993. *Tools, Language and Cognition in Human Evolution*. Cambridge University Press, Cambridge, U.K.

Gowlett, J.A.J. 1996. Mental abilities of early *Homo*: Elements of constraint and choice in rule systems. Pages 191–215 *in* P. Mellars & K. Gibson, eds., *Modeling the Early Human Mind*. McDonald Institute for Archaeological Research, Cambridge, U.K.

Grün, R. & C. Stringer. 1991. Electron spin resonance dating and the evolution of modern humans. *Archaeometry* 33:153-199.

Hahn, J. 1972. Aurignacian signs, pendants, and art objects in Central and Eastern Europe. *World Archaeol.* 3:252-266.

————. 1977. *Aurignacien: Das Altere Jungpaläolithikum in Mittel- und Osteuropa*. Fundamenta Series A9, Köln, Germany.

————. 1993. Aurignacian art in Central Europe. Pages 229–241 *in* H. Knecht, A. Pike-Tay & R. White, eds., *Before Lascaux: The Complex Record of the Early Upper Paleolithic*. CRC Press, Boca Raton.

Harpending, H., S. Sherry, A. Rogers, & M. Stoneking. 1993. The genetic structure of ancient human populations. *Curr. Anthropol.* 34:483–496.

Hayden, B. 1993. The cultural capacities of Neanderthals: A review and reevaluation. *Jour. Hum. Evol.* 24:113–146.

Hodder, I. 1982. *Symbols in Action: Ethnoarchaeological Studies of Material Culture*. Cambridge University Press, Cambridge, U.K.

Howell, F.C. 1996. Thoughts on the study and interpretation of the human fossil record. Pages 1–45 *in* W.E. Meikle, F.C. Howell, & N.G. Jablonski, eds., *Contemporary Issues in Human Evolution*. California Academy of Sciences, Memoir 21, San Francisco.

Humphrey, N. 1976. The social functions of intellect. Pages 303–317 *in* P.P.G. Bateson & R. A. Hinde, eds., *Growing Points in Ethology*. Cambridge University Press, Cambridge, U.K.

Isaac, G.Ll. 1972. Early phases of human behaviour: Models in Lower Paleolithic archaeology. Pages 167–199 *in* D.L. Clarke, ed., *Models in Archaeology*. Methuen, London, U.K.

Jochim, M. 1983. Paleolithic cave art in ecological perspective. Pages 212–219 *in* G.N. Bailey, ed., *Hunter-gatherer Economy in Prehistory: A European Perspective*. Cambridge University Press, Cambridge, U.K.

Klein, R.G. 1989. *The Human Career: Human Biological and Cultural Origins*. University of Chicago Press, Chicago.

Knecht, H. 1993. Splits and wedges: The techniques and technology of early Aurignacian antler working. Pages 137–162 *in* H. Knecht, A. Pike-Tay, & R. White, eds., *Before Lascaux: The Complex Record of the Early Upper Paleolithic*. CRC Press, Boca Raton.

Knecht, H., A. Pike-Tay, & R. White, R. eds. 1993. *Before Lascaux: The Complex Record of the Early Upper Paleolithic*. CRC Press, Boca Raton.

Knight, C.D. 1991. *Blood relations: Menstruation and the Origins of Culture*. Yale University Press, New Haven.

Knight, C., C. Power, & I. Watts. 1995. The human symbolic revolution: A Darwinian account. *Cambr. Archaeol. Jour.* 5:75–114.

Kozlowski, J.K. 1990. A multi-aspectual approach to the origins of the Upper Paleolithic in Europe. Pages 419–437 *in* P. Mellars, ed., *The Emergence of Modern Humans: an archaeological perspective*. Edinburgh University Press, Edinburgh.

Kozlowski, J.K. & S.K. Kozlowski. 1979. *Upper Paleolithic and Mesolithic in Europe: Taxonomy and Prehistory*. Polska Akademia Nauk, Cracow, Poland.

Krings, M., A. Stone, R.W. Schmitz, H. Krainitzki, M. Stoneking, & S. Pääbo. 1997. Neanderthal DNA sequences and the origin of modern humans. *Cell* 90:19–30.

Lahr, M.M., & R. Foley. 1994. Multiple dispersals and modern human origins. *Evol. Anthropol.* 3:48–60.

Lieberman, D.E. & J.J. Shea. 1994. Behavioral differences between archaic and modern humans in the Levantine Mousterian. *Amer. Anthropol.* 96:300–322.

Lieberman, P. 1989. The origins of some aspects of human language and cognition. Pages 391–414 *in* P. Mellars & C. Stringer, eds., *The Human Revolution: Behavioral and Biological Perspectives on the Origins of Modern Humans*. Princeton University Press, Princeton.

———. 1991. *Uniquely Human: The Evolution of Speech, Thought, and Selfless Behavior*. Harvard University Press, Cambridge.

Lourandos, H. 1996. *Continent of Hunter-Gatherers: New Perspectives in Australian Prehistory*. Cambridge University Press, Cambridge, U.K.

Marshack, A. 1991. *The Roots of Civilization*. Moyer Bell, Mount Kisco, New York.

Mellars, P.A. 1969. The chronology of Mousterian industries in the Perigord region of southwest France. *Proceed. Prehist. Soc.* 35:134–171.

———. 1973. The character of the Middle-Upper Paleolithic transition in southwest France. Pages 255–276 *in* C. Renfrew, ed., *The Explanation of Culture Change: Models in Prehistory*. Duckworth, London, U.K.

———. 1985. The ecological basis of social complexity in the Upper Paleolithic of southwestern France. Pages 271–297 *in* T.D. Price & J.A. Brown, eds., *Prehistoric Hunter-Gatherers: The Emergence of Cultural Complexity*. Academic Press, Orlando.

———. 1989a. Major issues in the emergence of modern humans. *Curr. Anthropol.* 30:349–385.

———. 1989b. Technological changes across the Middle-Upper Paleolithic transition: Technological, social, and cognitive perspectives. Pages 338–365 *in* P. Mellars & C. Stringer, eds., *The Human Revolution: Behavioral and Biological Perspectives on the Origins of Modern Humans*. Princeton University Press, Princeton.

————. 1991. Cognitive changes and the emergence of modern humans in Europe. *Cambr. Archaeol. Jour.* 1:63–76.

————. 1992. Archaeology and the population-dispersal hypothesis of modern human origins in Europe. Pages 225–234 *in* M. Aitken, C.B. Stringer, & P.A. Mellars, eds., *The Origin of Modern Humans and the Impact of Chronometric Dating*. Royal Society (Philosophical Transactions of the Royal Society, series B, 337, no. 1280), London, U.K.

————. 1996a. *The Neanderthal Legacy: An Archaeological Perspective from Western Europe*. Princeton University Press, Princeton.

————. 1996b. Symbolism, language and the Neanderthal mind. Pages 15–32 *in* P. Mellars & K. Gibson, eds., *Modeling the Early Human Mind*. McDonald Institute for Archaeological Research, Cambridge, U.K.

————. 1996c. The emergence of biologically modern populations in Europe: A social and cognitive 'revolution'? Pages 179–201 *in* W.G. Runciman, J. Maynard Smith, & R.I. Dunbar, eds., *The Evolution of Social Behaviour Patterns in Primates and Man*. Oxford University Press (Proceedings of the British Academy, vol. 88), Oxford, U.K.

Mithen, S. 1990. *Thoughtful Foragers: A Study of Prehistoric Decision Making*. Cambridge University Press, Cambridge, U.K.

————. 1996a. *The Prehistory of the Mind: A Search for the Origins of Art, Religion and Science*. Thames & Hudson, London, U.K.

————. 1996b. Domain-specific intelligence and the Neanderthal mind. Pages 217–229 *in* P. Mellars & K. Gibson, eds., *Modelling the Early Human Mind*. McDonald Institute for Archaeological Research, Cambridge, U.K.

Mussi, M. 1992. *Popoli e Civilta' dell'Italia Antica. Volume Decimo: Il Paleolitico e il Mesolitico in Italia*. Biblioteca di Storia Patria, Bologna, Italy.

Nitecki, M.H. & D.V. Nitecki, eds. 1994. *Origins of Anatomically Modern Humans*. Plenum Press, New York.

Noble, W. & I. Davidson. 1996. *Human Evolution, Language and Mind: A Psychological and Archaeological Inquiry*. Cambridge University Press, Cambridge, U.K.

Oswalt, W.H. 1976. *An Anthropological Analysis of Food-getting Technology*. John Wiley, New York.

Otte. M. 1981. *Le Gravettien en Europe Centrale*. Dissertationes Archaeologicae Gandenses, No. 20, Bruges, Belgium.

Passingham, R.E., 1989. The origins of human intelligence. Pages 123–136 *in* R. Durant, ed., *Human Origins*. Clarendon Press, London, U.K.

Peterson, N., ed. 1976. *Tribes and Boundaries in Australia*. Australian Institute for Aboriginal Studies, Canberra, U.K.

Pfeiffer, J.E. 1982. *The Creative Explosion: An Inquiry into the Origins of Art and Religion*. Harper & Row, New York.

Pinker, S. 1994. *The Language Instinct: The New Science of Language and Mind*. Penguin, London, U.K.

Price, T.D. & J.A. Brown, eds. 1985. *Prehistoric Hunter-Gatherers: The Emergence of Cultural Complexity*. Academic Press, Orlando.

Ragir, S. 1985. Retarded development: The evolutionary mechanism underlying the emergence of language. *Jour. Mind Behav.* 6:451–468.

Renfrew, C. 1996. The sapient behaviour paradox: How to test for potential? Pages 11–14 *in* P. Mellars & K. Gibson, eds., *Modelling the Early Human Mind*. McDonald Institute for Archaeological Research, Cambridge, U.K.

Rodseth, L., R.W. Wrangham, A.M. Harrigan, & B.B. Smuts. 1991. The human community as a primate society. *Curr. Anthropol.* 32:221–254.

Sackett, J. 1988. The Mousterian and its aftermath: A view from the Upper Paleolithic. Pages 413–426 *in* H.L. Dibble & A. Montet-White, eds., *Upper Pleistocene Prehistory of Western Eurasia*. University Museum of Pennsylvania, Monograph 54, Philadelphia.

Schick, K.D. & N. Toth. 1993. *Making Silent Stones Speak: Human Evolution and the Dawn of Technology*. Weidenfeld & Nicolson, London, U.K.

Shennan, S. 1996. Social inequality and the transmission of cultural traditions in forager societies. Pages 365–379 *in* J. Steele & S. Shennan, eds., *The Archaeology of Human Ancestry*. Routledge, London, U.K.

Singer, R. & J. Wymer. 1982. *The Middle Stone Age at Klasies River Mouth in South Africa*. University of Chicago Press, Chicago.

Smith, P.E.L. 1964. The Solutrean culture. *Sci. Amer.* 211:86–94.

———. 1966. *Le Solutréen en France*. Delmas, Bordeaux, France.

Soffer, O., 1994. Ancestral lifeways in Eurasia — the Middle and Upper Paleolithic records. Pages 101–109 *in* M.H. Nitecki & D.V. Nitecki, eds., *Origins of Anatomically Modern Humans*. Plenum Press, New York.

Sonneville-Bordes, D. de. 1960. *Le Paléolithique Supérieur en Pérgord*. Delmas, Bordeaux, France.

Stoneking, M., S.T. Sherry, A.J. Redd, & L. Vigilant. 1992. New approaches to dating suggest a recent age for the human DNA ancestor. Pages 167–176 *in* M. Aitken, C.B. Stringer & P.A. Mellars, eds., *The Origin of Modern Humans and the Impact of Chronometric Dating*. Royal Society (Philosophical Transactions of the Royal Society, series B, 337, no. 1280), London, U.K.

Straus, L.G. & C.W. Heller. 1988. Explorations in the twilight zone: The Upper Paleolithic of Vasco-Cantabrian Spain and Gascogny. Pages 97–134 *in* J.F. Hoffecker & C.A. Wolf, eds., *The Early Upper Paleolithic: evidence from Europe and the Near East*. British Archaeological Reports S437, Oxford, U.K.

Stringer, C. & C. Gamble. 1993. *In Search of the Neanderthals: Solving the Puzzle of Human Origins*. Thames & Hudson, London, U.K.

Stringer, C. & R. McKie. 1996. *African Exodus: The Origins of Modern Humanity*. Jonathan Cape, London, U.K.

Taborin, Y. 1993. Shells of the French Aurignacian and Perigordian. Pages 211–229 *in* H. Knecht, A. Pike-Tay, & R. White, eds., *Before Lascaux: The Complex Record of the Early Upper Paleolithic*. CRC Press, Boca Raton.

Tishkoff, S.A., E. Dietzsch, W. Speed, A.J. Pakstis, J.R. Kidd, K. Cheung, B. Bonné Tamir, A.S. Santachiara-Benerecetti, P. Moral, M. Krings, S. Pääbo, E. Watson, N. Risch, T. Jenkins & K.K. Kidd. 1996. Global patterns of linkage disequilibrium at the CD4 locus and modern human origins. *Science* 271:1380–1387.

Tooby, J. & L. Cosmides. 1992. The psychological foundations of culture. Pages 19–136 *in* J.H. Barkow, L. Cosmides, & J. Tooby, eds., *The Adapted Mind*. Oxford University Press, Oxford, U.K.

Van Andel, T. & P.C. Tzedakis. 1996. Palaeolithic landscapes of Europe and environs, 150,000-25,000 years ago. *Quat. Sci. Rev.* 15:481–500.

Vandermeersch, B. 1970. Une sépulture moustérien avec offrandes découverte dans la grotte de Qafzeh. *Comptes Rendus de l'Académie des Sciences de Paris* 270:298–301.

———. 1976. Les sépultures néanderthaliennes. Pages 725–727 *in* H. de Lumley, ed., *La Préhistoire Française*. Centre National de la Recherche Scientifique, Paris, France.

Wiessner, P. 1983. Style and social information in Kalahari San projectile points. *Amer. Antiquity* 48:253–276.

———. 1984. Reconsidering the behavioral basis for style: a case study among the Kalahari San. *Jour. Anthropol. Archaeol.* 3:190–234.

Whallon, R. 1989. Elements of cultural change in the later Palaeolithic. Pages 433–454 *in* P. Mellars & C. Stringer, eds., *The Human Revolution: Behavioral and Biological Perspectives on the Origins of Modern Humans*. Princeton University Press, Princeton.

White, R. 1989. Production complexity and standardization in early Aurignacian bead and pendant manufacture: evolutionary implications. Pages 366–390 *in* P. Mellars & C. Stringer, eds., *The Human Revolution: Behavioral and Biological Perspectives on the Origins of Modern Humans*. Princeton University Press, Princeton.

———. 1993. Technological and social dimensions of "Aurignacian-age" body ornaments across Europe. Pages 277–300 *in* H. Knecht, A. Pike-Tay, & R. White, eds., *Before Lascaux: The Complex Record of the Early Upper Paleolithic*. CRC Press, Boca Raton.

Wolpoff, M.H., A.G. Thorne, F.H. Smith, D.W. Frayer, & G.G. Pope. 1994. Multiregional evolution: a worldwide source for modern human populations. Pages 175–199 *in* M.H. Nitecki, & D.V. Nitecki, eds., *Origins of Anatomically Modern Humans*. Plenum Press, New York.

A 2399-903

VAN NESS NORTH
3

JAN 7 P 2:28

ISE BEFORE TIME ABOVE

 RETAIN AS
PROOF OF PAYMENT

**TRANSFER /
FARE RECEIPT**

WELCOME

Tickets issued
machines are va
time shown and r
as transfers to oth

For faster loading,
sent face up with ti
showing.

Not valid on cab

Buying or selling
prohibited by P
Section 640.

MUNI CRIME
(415) 671-3179 (
IN EMERGENCY

Commendations & C
Passenger Service (415

For general inforr
(415) 673-MUNI.

THANK YOU FOR YOUR

The Evolution of the Human Language Faculty

Steven Pinker
Department of Brain and Cognitive Sciences
Massachusetts Institute of Technology
Cambridge, MA 02139

Language is the remarkable faculty by which humans convey thoughts to one another by means of a highly structured signal. Language works by two principles: A dictionary of memorized symbols, that is, words, and a set of generative rules organized into several subsystems, that is, grammar. The machinery of language appears to have been designed to encode and decode propositional information for the purpose of sharing it with others. Language is universally complex and develops reliably throughout the species, partly independently of general intelligence. I suggest that language is an adaptation for sharing information. It fits with many other features of our zoologically distinctive "informavore" niche, in which people acquire, share, and apply knowledge of how the world works to outsmart plants, animals, and each other.

If an alien biologist studying the human species were to observe us in this room today, it would be struck by the fact that you are sitting quietly doing nothing but listening to a man make noises as he exhales. This remarkable habit of our species is called language. You are listening to my exhaling noises because I have coded information into some of the acoustic properties of that noise which your brains have the ability to decode. By this means I am able to transfer ideas from inside my head to inside your head.

In this paper I will say a few words about the design of the human language faculty — the tricks behind the ability to transfer information by making noise — and about whether language is an adaptation, and if so, what it is for. (For more detailed discussion of many of these points, see Pinker 1994.)

Reprinted with minor changes from Pinker, S. 1997. Language as a psychological adaptation. Pages 162-180 *in* G.R. Bock & G. Cardew, eds., *Characterizing Human Psychological Adaptations*. Ciba Foundation Symposium 208. Wiley, Chichester, U.K., by permission of the author and the Ciba Foundation.

The Design of Human Language

What is the secret behind my ability to cause you to think specific thoughts by means of the vocal channel? There is not one secret, but two, and they were identified in the 19th century by continental linguists.

Words

The first principle was articulated by Ferdinand de Saussure and lies behind the mental dictionary, our finite memorized list of words. A word is an arbitrary symbol, a connection between a signal and an idea shared by all members of the community. The word *duck* doesn't look like a duck, walk like a duck or quack like a duck. However, I can use it to convey the idea of a duck because we all have, in our developmental history, formed the same connection between the sound and the meaning. Therefore, I can bring the idea to mind virtually instantaneously simply by making that noise. If instead I had to shape the signal to evoke the thought in your mind using some sensible connection between its form and its content, every word would require the amusing but inefficient contortions of a game of Charades.

The symbols underlying words are bidirectional. Generally if I can say something, I can understand it, and *vice versa*. When children learn words, their tongues are not molded into the right shape by parents, and they do not need to go through a process of being rewarded for successive approximations to the target sound for every word they learn. Instead, children have an ability upon hearing somebody else use a word to know that they in turn can use it to that person or to a third party and expect to be understood.

Another noteworthy feature of the mental dictionary is its size. One can use dictionary sampling techniques to estimate how many independent memorizations must have taken place to install a typical adult vocabulary. For example, if you take the largest dictionary you can find, pick the third word down on the right hand side of every tenth page, put the word in a multiple-choice test say, correct for guessing, and then multiply the performance on the test by the size of the dictionary, you obtain estimates for a typical high school student of about 60,000 independent words, probably twice that number for a highly literate high school student. The learning rate for the smaller estimate works out to be about one word every 90 minutes, starting at the age of one. Considering that every one of these words is as arbitrary as a telephone number or a date in history, it is remarkable that children pick one up every hour and a half, at the same time as they are struggling over multiplication tables, the date of the Treaty of Versailles, and so on.

Grammar

Of course we don't just learn individual words. We combine them into strings when we talk, and that leads to the second trick behind language, grammar. The principle behind grammar was articulated by Wilhelm von Humboldt as "the infinite use of finite media." Inside everyone's head there is a finite algorithm — it has to be finite because the head is finite — with the ability to generate an infinite number of potential sentences, each of which corresponds to a distinct thought. For example, our knowledge of English incorporates rules that say "a sentence may be composed of a noun phrase (subject) and a verb phrase (object)" and "a verb phrase may be composed of a verb, a noun phrase (object), and a sentence (complement)." That pair of rules is [recursive]: an element is introduced on the right hand side of one rule which is also on the left hand side of the other rule, creating the possibility of a loop that could generate sentences of any size, such as "I think that she thinks that he said that I wonder whether ...." We can generate an infinite number of sentences, and each sentence expresses a distinct thought. Therefore this system gives us the ability to put an unlimited number of distinct thoughts into words, and other people to interpret the string of words to recover the thoughts.

Grammar can be thought of as a discrete combinatorial system, which can be opposed to a blending system. In a blending system all the possibilities that you get when you combine the ingredients lie on a continuum between the two endpoints. For example, if you mix red paint and white paint you obtain various degrees of pink paint, which differ in an analogue fashion. In a discrete combinatorial system, such as DNA, atoms, molecules, and sentences, each one of the combinations can be qualitatively different from the other combinations and from the ingredients. Therefore, there is an infinite number of thoughts, but the set is infinite in a discrete way as opposed to a continuous way.

Grammar can express a remarkable range of thoughts because our knowledge of languages resides in an algorithm that combines abstract symbols, such as noun and verb, as opposed to concrete concepts, such as man and dog or eater and eaten. This gives us an ability to talk about all kinds of wild and wonderful ideas. We can talk about a dog biting a man, or, as in the journalist's definition of "news," a man biting a dog. We can talk about aliens landing at Harvard. We can talk about the universe beginning with a big bang, or the ancestors of native Americans immigrating to the continent over a land bridge from Asia during an Ice Age, or Michael Jackson marrying Elvis's daughter. All kinds of novel ideas can be communicated because our knowledge of language is couched in abstract symbols like "noun" and "verb" which can embrace a vast set of concepts, and then can be combined freely into an even vaster set of propositions. How vast? In principle it is infinite; in practice it can be crudely estimated by assessing the number of word choices possible at each point in a sentence (roughly, 10) and raising it to a power corresponding to the maximum length of a sentence a person is likely to produce and understand, say, 20. The number is 10^{20} or about a hundred million trillion sentences.

Let me say a bit more about the design of the human grammatical system. Grammar is not just a single pair of rules, as I listed above, but hundreds or thousands of rules, which fall into a number of subsystems. The most prominent is syntax, the component of language that combines words into phrases and sentences. One of the tools of syntax is word order. That is the tool that allows us to distinguish *Man bites dog* from *Dog bites man*. Order is the first thing people think of when they think about syntax, but in fact it is a relatively superficial manifestation; there are complex principles that underlie its ability to convey ideas.

Far more important than linear word order is constituency. A sentence has a hierarchical structure. It can be represented as a bracketed string of phrases embedded within phrases, which allow us to convey complex propositions of ideas embedded inside ideas. A simple demonstration of the brain's ability to parse sentences into hierarchical phrase structures is an (unintentionally) ambiguous sentence published in *TV Guide: On tonight's program Dr. Ruth will discuss sex with Dick Cavett*. We have a single string of words in a particular order, but it has two very different meanings. The intended meaning was that Dick Cavett is who you discuss sex with, and the alternative meaning is that sex with Dick Cavett is what you discussed. In this particular sentence they are, unfortunately, expressed by the same string of words; the different interpretations correspond to the different phrase structure bracketings our brain can impose on that string. Thankfully, not all sentences are as blatantly ambiguous as that one, and the brain's ability to compute phrase structure is put to use in recovering the single meaning that the speaker intended. Much as in other symbolic systems that encode logical information, such as arithmetic, propositional calculus, and computer programming, it is important in linguistic communication to get the parentheses right, and that's what phrase structure is for.

Syntax also involves predicate-argument structure, the component of language that encodes the information that a logician would express as a predicate, that is, a relationship among a set of participants, and its arguments, that is, the particular participants in a given instance of that relationship. In particular, what your grammar school teacher called the predicate of the sentence, namely the verb, is similar in many ways to what a logician would call a predicate. To understand a sentence you cannot merely pay attention to the order of words, or even just group them. You have to look up information associated with the predicate. A simple demonstration the pair of sentences *Man fears dog* and *Man frightens dog*. The word *man* is the subject of both of these sentences, but the semantic role that *man* is playing in the first sentence is different from the role it is playing in the second sentence: In one case the man is causing the fear; in the other the man is being affected by fear. That shows that in understanding a sentence you have to look up information stored with the mental dictionary entry of the verb and see whether it says "my subject is the one doing the fearing" or "my subject is the one causing the fear."

A fourth trick of syntax is the operation called the transformation, which is associated most strongly with Noam Chomsky's theory of transformational grammar. After you have generated a hierarchical tree structure into which the words of a sentence are plugged, a further set of operations can mangle the order of words in precise ways. For example, the sentence *Dog is bitten by man* contains the verb bite, *which* ordinarily requires a direct object. But in this sentence the object is missing from its customary location; it has been moved to the front of the sentence. This gives us a means of shifting the emphasis and the quantification of a given set of participants in a relationship. The sentence *Man bites dog* and *Dog is bitten by man* both express the same information about who did what to whom — a man does the biting, a dog gets bitten — but one of them is a comment about the man and the other is a comment about the dog. Similarly, sentences in which a phrase is replaced by a [wh]-word and moved to the front of a sentence, such as *Who did the dog bite?*, allow the speaker to seek the identity of one of the participants in a given interaction. Transformations, therefore, give us a layer of meaning above and beyond who did what to whom. That layer emphasizes or seeks information about one participant or another, while keeping the actual event that one is talking about constant.

Syntax, for all that complexity, is only one component of grammar. All languages have a second combinatorial system, morphology, in which bits of words are assembled to produce whole words. In English we don't have much morphology, compared with other languages, but we have some. The noun *duck* comes in two forms — *duck* and *ducks* — and the verb *quack* in four — *quack*, *quacks*, *quacked*, and *quacking*. In other languages morphology plays a much greater role. In Latin, for example, there is a rich inflectional system which plays an important role in expression. By placing suffixes onto the ends of nouns, one can convey information about who did what to whom, allowing one to scramble the left-to-right order of the words for emphasis or style. For example, *Canis hominem mordet* and *Hominem canis mordet* have the same non-newsworthy meaning, and *Homo canem mordet* and *Canem homo mordet* have the same newsworthy meaning.

In addition to syntax and morphology, language comprises a third combinatorial system — a third layer of assembly of elements into larger elements by rules, called phonology. The rules of phonology govern the sound pattern of a language. In no language do people form words by associating them directly with articulatory gestures like a movement of the tongue or lips. Instead, a fixed set of articulatory gestures is combined into sequences, each sequence defining a word. The combinations are governed by phonological rules that people have to acquire as they acquire a language. In English, for example, we know that *bluck* is not a word but could be a word, whereas *nguck* is not a word and could not be a word because the English rules of word formation don't allow the consonant *ng* at the beginning. In other languages, *ng* can be placed there. Interestingly, whereas syntax and morphology are semantically compositional, that is, you can predict the meaning of the whole by the meanings of the elements and the way they are combined, this is not true of phonology. You cannot predict the meaning of *duck* from the meaning of *d*, the meaning of *u*, and the meaning of *k*. The combinatorial system called phonology simply allows us to have large vocabularies, for example, 100,000 words, without having to pair each one of them with a different simple noise coming out of the mouth.

Phonology also consists of a set of adjustment rules which, after the words are defined and combined into phrases, smooth out the sequence of articulatory gestures to make them easier to pronounce and comprehend. One of those rules in English causes us to pronounce the same morpheme -*ed* for the past tense in three different ways depending on what it is attached to. In *jogged* it is pronounced as *d*. In *walked* it is pronounced as a *t*, thanks to a rule that keeps the consonants at the end of a word either all voiced (larynx buzzing) or all unvoiced. And in *patted* the suffix is pronounced with the neutral schwa vowel before it, thanks to a rule that inserts a vowel to separate two *d*-like sounds. Therefore, even though the actual morpheme is the same in all cases, that is, *d*, there are rules that fiddle with the pronunciation pattern before it is articulated. These adjustments are not just peoples' effort to be clear, or for that matter their tendency to be lazy, as they put words together. There is a set of regulations for each language that dictate when you are allowed to be lazy and when you are not, and they are partly arbitrary in that you acquire them as you acquire the sound pattern of a language. (An accent is what happens when someone applies the phonological adjustment rules of one language to the content of another language.) Phonological rules have the function of helping people achieve a mixture of clarity and ease of pronunciation, but they are a distinct part of one's knowledge of language.

Interfaces of Language With Other Parts of the Mind

Grammar is only one component of language. It has to look toward the rest of the mind in three different directions. Grammar has to be connected to the ear, so that we can understand; to the mouth, so that we can articulate; and to the rest of the mind, so that we can say sensible things in the context of a conversation. Each requires an interface.

The first interface is the speech articulation or articulatory phonetic system. One of the salient properties of this system is the actual anatomy of the vocal tract, which seems to have evolved in the human lineage in the service of the language. Darwin pointed to the fact that every mouthful of food we swallow has to pass over the trachea, with some chance of getting lodged in it and causing death by choking. The human vocal tract has a low larynx by mammalian standards; this placement compromises a number of physiological functions but allows us to articulate a large range of vowel sounds. Because our larynx is so low in the throat it gives room for the tongue to move both back and forth and up and down independently. This defines a two-dimensional space in which the tongue can move. Because there are two resonant cavities, defined by the position of the tongue with respect to the throat, on one hand, and the mouth, on the other, we can produce a two-dimensional space of vowel sounds, which multiplies out the number of distinct discriminable signals we can articulate. One can argue that given the physiological cost, that is, the risk of death by choking, there must have been a corresponding benefit in our evolutionary history, presumably the benefit of rapid, expressive communication.

The second interface is speech comprehension. Information being received by the ear has to be unpacked into a meaning. One of the remarkable features of speech comprehension is the way in which the brain can unpack a stream of sound into its component words, which are not physically demarcated in the sound stream by little silences analogous to the small spaces that separate words on a printed page. When we hear language as a string of words we are the victims of an illusion. We realize this only when we hear speech in another language: to our ears it sounds like a continuous ribbon of sound, which is exactly what it is, physically speaking. Another demonstration bringing this feat to our attention is a kind of wordplay seen in doggerel such as "Mairzey doats and dozey doats" (Mares eat oats and does eat oats) and "Fuzzy Wuzzy was a bear," which are designed to exploit the fact that speech is not a discrete chain of words separated by silence.

Another remarkable feature of speech comprehension is the rate at which information can be conveyed. A rapid talker can convey about 40 phonemes per second, and even a more leisurely talker can reach 10 to 20 phonemes per second. Twenty cycles per second is the lower limit of pitch perception in humans. We hear 20 beats per second not as 20 rapid events but as a low tone or a buzz. Clearly, when we are listening to speech at 25 phonemes per second we are not registering 25 separate auditory events, because that is neurologically impossible. There must be some sort of multiplexing or compression of the information, in which the phonemes are superimposed in the process of speaking and the brain has to unpack them in the process of understanding.

Finally, language has an interface with more general inference systems. The decoding of the literal information conveyed by words and grammar is just the first step of a long chain of inference by which we try to guess what the speaker wants us to think he or she is trying to say. We engage in this process of inference even in understanding the simple sentences. A nice example from the linguist Jim McCawley shows the knowledge we must apply to something as simple as assigning referents to pronouns such as *he* and *she*. Imagine a dialogue in which Marsha says "I'm leaving" and John says "Who is he"? We all know who "he" is, not by any information that is explicitly encoded in the sentence, but by our knowledge about human behavior. Those expectations are brought to bear in understanding a sentence, in conjunction with the particular rules of grammar.

Is Language an Adaptation?

With that summary of the design of the human language faculty in mind, we can now turn to the question: Is language an adaptation? Darwin wrote, "Man has an instinctive tendency to speak, as we see in the babble of our young children, while no child has an instinctive tendency to bake, brew or write." This is probably the first statement that human language is an adaptation. What are the alternatives, and what is the evidence?

One alternative is that language is not an adaptation itself, but is a manifestation of more general cognitive abilities, some form of "general intelligence," in which case general intelligence would be the adaptation, not language. There is a reasonable amount of evidence against this possibility.

First, language is universal across societies and across all neurologically normal people within a society. There may be technologically primitive peoples, but there are no primitive languages. And the language of uneducated, working class, and rural speakers has been found to be systematic and rule-governed, though the rules may belong to a dialect that did not have the good fortune of becoming the standard dialect of Britain and its former colonies.

Second, languages conform to a universal design. The languages of the highlands of New Guinea, for example, use computational machinery that is identical to that described earlier in this paper, even though that machinery was motivated by an examination of English and other European languages.

A third kind of evidence was alluded to by Darwin: the ontogenetic development of language. There is a uniform sequence of stages that children pass through all over the world. That sequence culminates in mastery of the local language, despite the computational difficulty of programming a computational system to take in a finite sample of sentences from a couple of speakers (the child's parents) and induce a grammar for the infinite rest of the language. Moreover, children's speech patterns, including their errors, are highly systematic, and often conform to linguistic universals for which there was no direct evidence in parents' speech.

A fourth kind of evidence also comes from the study of language acquisition. If children are thrown together without a model language, such as in a multilingual plantation or, if the children are deaf, a school that does not have people using sign language, the children will develop a systematic, rule-governed language of their own, a phenomenon called creolization.

A fifth kind of evidence is that language and general intelligence, to the extent we can make sense of that term, seem to be doubly dissociable in neurological and genetic disorders. In aphasias and in a developmental syndrome (probably genetic in origin) called Specific Language Impairment, intelligent people can have extreme difficulties speaking and understanding. Conversely, in what clinicians informally call "chatterbox syndromes," severely retarded children may talk a stream of fully grammatical English but with a content that is highly childlike or is confabulated, bearing no relation to the world.

A different alternative to the hypothesis that language is an adaptation is the possibility that language indeed is a separate system from general intelligence, but that it evolved by nonselectionist mechanisms. Perhaps, on this view, language evolved all at once as the product of a macromutation, or as a byproduct of some other evolutionary development such as evolving a large head. The main reason to doubt this theory is the standard argument for the operation of natural selection, the argument from adaptive complexity. The information processing circuitry necessary to produce, comprehend and learn language must involve a great deal of organization and detail. As with other complex biological systems that accomplish improbable feats, this circuitry is unlikely to have evolved by something as crude as a single mutation or some other evolutionary force that is insensitive to what the circuit accomplishes.

What Did Language Evolve For?

If language is an adaptation, what is it an adaptation for? Note that asking this question is different from asking what language is typically *used* for, especially what it is used for at present. The question concerns the engineering design of language and the extent to which it informs us about the selective pressures that shaped it.

What is the machinery of language trying to accomplish? The system looks as if it was put together to encode and decode digital propositional information — who did what to whom, what is true of what, when, where and why — into a signal that can be conveyed from one person to another.

It is not difficult to think of why it would have been a good thing for a species with the rest of our characteristics to evolve the ability to do this (Pinker 1997). The structures of grammar are well suited to conveying information about technology, such as which two things should be put together to produce a third thing; about the local environment, such as where things are and which people did what to whom; and about one's own intentions, such as "If you do this, I will do that," which convey relationships of exchange and of dominance, as in threats.

Gathering and exchanging information of this kind is, in turn, integral to the larger niche that modern *Homo sapiens* has filled, which George Miller has called the informavore niche and which John Tooby and Irven DeVore previously called the cognitive niche (Tooby & DeVore 1987). Tooby and DeVore have assembled a theory that tries to explain the list of properties of the human species that a biologist would consider zoologically unusual, such as our extensive manufacture of and dependence on complex tools, our wide range of habitats and diets, our long childhoods and long lives, our hypersociality, and our division into groups or cultures each with a set of distinctive local variations in behavior. Their explanation is that the human lifestyle is a consequence of a specialization for overcoming the evolutionary fixed defenses of plants and animals by cause-and-effect reasoning, which is driven by intuitive theories about various domains of the world, such as objects, forces, paths, places, manners, states, substances, hidden biochemical essences, and other people's beliefs and desires.

The information captured in these intuitive theories is reminiscent of the information that the machinery of grammar is designed to convert into strings of noises. It is probably not a coincidence that what is special about humans is that we outsmart other animals and plants by cause-and-effect reasoning, and language seems to be a way of converting information about cause-and-effect and action into a signal.

An unusual feature of information is that it can be duplicated without loss. If I give you a fish, I don't have the fish, as we know from sayings like "you can't eat your cake and have it." Information, however, *can* be both eaten and had: If I tell you how to fish, it is not the case that I now lack the knowledge of how to fish because I've given it away to you; we can both have it. There is a brilliant, eccentric computer programmer associated with MIT, Richard Stallman, who started a free software foundation based on the idea that no one should charge for software. While it's perfectly reasonable, he argues, for a baker to charge for bread, since there's only a finite amount of flour and once it is given to someone then someone else cannot have it. But once software is developed and can be copied, Stallman argues, there is no reason that it should not be free. If it is given to one person, that does *not* mean that someone else cannot have it (with the exception of the floppy disk itself).

Tooby and DeVore (1987) have pointed out that in a species like ours that lives on information, it is quite natural that in conjunction with evolving the ability to gather this information we evolved a means to exchange it. Having language multiplies the benefit of knowledge. Knowledge is not only useful to oneself as a way of figuring out, for example, how to build snares to catch rabbits, but it is also useful as a trade good: I can exchange it with somebody else at a low cost to myself and hope to get something in return. It can also lower the original acquisition cost. I can learn about how to catch a rabbit from someone else's trial and error; I don't have to go through it myself.

Language, therefore, fits with other features of the informavore niche. The zoologically unusual features of *Homo sapiens* can be united by the idea that humans have evolved an ability to encode information about the causal structure of the world and to share it among themselves. Our hypersociality makes sense because information is a particularly good commodity of exchange that makes it worth people's while to hang out together. Our long childhood is an apprenticeship — before we go out in the world, we spend a lot of time learning what everyone else around us has figured out already. The existence of culture can be seen as a kind of pool of local expertise. Many traditions develop locally because many of the requirements to deal with the various aspects of the world have been acquired by other people, resulting in a network of information sharing that is close to what sociologists and anthropologists have called "culture." Humans have long lifespans because once you've had an expensive education you might as well make the most out of it by having a long lifespan during which the expertise can be put to use. Humans inhabit a wide range of habitats because we don't have knowledge that is highly specialized, such as how to catch a rabbit; our knowledge is more abstract, such as how living things work and how objects bump into each other. That machinery for construing the world can be applied to many kinds of environments; it is not specific to a particular ecosystem.

People have occasionally raised objections to the hypothesis that language is an adaptation for sharing information. One objection is that organisms are competitors, so sharing information is in fact costly by virtue of the advantages it gives to one's competitors. If I teach someone to fish, they may overfish the local lake, leaving no fish for me. The argument, however, just boils down to the standard problem of the difficulties facing the evolution of cooperation or altruism, and the solution in the case of language is the same. By sharing information with our kin, we help copies of our genes inside those kin, and when it comes to sharing information with nonrelatives, if we ensure that we inform only those people who return the favor, we both gain the benefits of trade. Certainly we do use our faculties of social cognition to ration our conversation with those with whom we have established a nonexploitative relationship; hence the expression "to be on speaking terms."

A second objection is that language may be used to deceive, so perhaps language evolved as a means of manipulation rather than as means of communication. The answer to the objection is, once again, that language surely coevolved with our faculties of social cognition. We apply those faculties as we listen to others; we are constantly vigilant for whether we are being lied to. And I find it hard to imagine any coherent account by which language evolved to allow us to manipulate others. Unlike signals with the physiological power to manipulate another organism directly, such as loud noises or chemicals, the signals of language are impotent unless the recipient actively applies complicated neural machinery to decode them. It is impossible to use language to manipulate someone who doesn't understand the language, so if language is an adaptation to manipulate others, how could it have gotten off the ground? What would have been the evolutionary incentive for the designated targets to evolve those exquisitely complex mental algorithms for unpacking the speech wave into words and assembling them into trees? Like a shop owner who makes sure he is not around when the gangster selling "protection" comes by, or a negotiator who remains incommunicado until a deadline passes, hominids in the presence of the first linguistic manipulators would have done best by refusing to allow their nascent language systems to evolve further, and language evolution would have been over before it began.

Literature Cited

Pinker, S. 1994. *The Language Instinct*. Harper Collins, New York.
———.1997. *How the Mind Works*. Norton, New York.
Tooby, J. & I. DeVore. 1987. The reconstruction of hominid evolution through strategic modeling. Pages 183–237 *in* W.G. Kinzey, ed., *The Evolution of Human Behavior: Primate Models*. SUNY Press, New York.

The Origin and Dispersal of Languages: Linguistic Evidence

Johanna Nichols
Department of Slavic Languages and Literatures
University of California
Berkeley, CA 94720

Tracing the descent of languages and reconstructing language families has produced some of the great achievements of linguistic science in the 19th and 20th centuries, including classification of most of the world's languages as well as detailed linguistic reconstructions and fairly precise dates of origin for great language families such as Indo-European, Uralic, Semitic, Bantu, Dravidian, Chinese, Algonquian, Mayan, Austronesian, and others. Specific cultural reconstructions follow from reconstructed vocabulary and dates, and consequently many of these families have been rather securely linked to places of origin and some even to archeological cultures. But linguistic descent cannot be traced back more than about 10,000 to 12,000 years at the very most, and secure reconstruction has not succeeded beyond about 6000 years, since regular grammar change and vocabulary loss gradually remove the critical evidence for ancestral vocabulary and grammar and the diagnostics that prove relatedness. Though this fade-out threshold is an absolute obstacle to reconstructing the ultimate ancestor(s) of the world's languages, it can be turned to advantage, for it provides a temporal threshold enabling linguists to identify descent lineages of an approximately identical absolute age. This in turn makes possible various kinds of comparison which, together with some basic principles of linguistic geography, yield information on the geography and time frame of ancient migrations and dispersals. The resultant picture, though still spare and approximate, is much richer than a wordlist and a family tree, which are all one could hope to gain from tracing descent far back.

Happily for present purposes, so little is known about the origin and dispersal of human language that everything we know can be outlined, at least in general form, in a single article. Let us begin with the notion of language family. There are about 6000 different languages spoken on Earth, and in the century and a half since the relevant comparative methods were developed linguists have succeeded in working out a genetic classification of almost all of them — rough and provisional in some cases but refined and precise in most.[1] The 6000 languages fall into about 300 families, which further comparative and descriptive work may eventually succeed in reducing to about 200 lineages. These families vary in their sizes and ages, but each is genetically discrete, and the oldest ones that we can trace are generally in the range of about 6000

years old. Descent of course goes back farther, but traceable descent fades out rapidly. This is because languages gradually change over time, and after a few millennia
the kind of evidence that can prove family relatedness, or help reconstruct the ancestral language, erodes beyond recognition. An average rate of vocabulary loss from a
standard word list of 100 or 200 items has been computed at about 20% per millennium, and dates of separation can be calculated for pairs of languages by determining
the number of cognate items they share from that list. (This technique is known as
glottochronology. For a recent textbook presentation see Trask 1996:361; for a refinement that produces remarkably accurate estimates of time depth, Embleton 1986,
1991.) After 6000 years of separation, two languages are expected to exhibit only 7%
shared cognates; and 7% represents the lowest number of resemblant items that can
safely be considered distinct from chance (for the latter figure see Nichols,
submitted). Hence the 6000-year age of the oldest securely reconstructable language
families is also the age after which, on binary tests, the incidence of cognates slips below the level of significance.[2]

Thus, though there are a few exceptions (some mentioned below), 6000 years can
be taken as a rule-of-thumb average for the oldest securely traceable language families. Now, anatomically modern humanity is about 100,000 years old, and, since the
modern anatomy includes a speech tract dedicated to speech production and aural and
cognitive capacities dedicated to speech decoding, it is safe to estimate that human
language as we know it is at least 100,000 years old. Six thousand years just barely
scratches the surface of this language prehistory. Therefore, there is no hope of recovering information about language origins by tracing linguistic descent.

Furthermore, even if descent could be traced back beyond 6000 or so years, much
important information would be missing. It is well known that many of the world's
language families have gone extinct. From the ancient Near East alone, in just the last
two to three thousand years Sumerian, Elamite, the Hurrian-Urartean line, and Hattic
have vanished without descendants or demonstrable kin. There is no reason to doubt
that extinction has always gone on, usually caused by language shift (for this term see
again note 1). Therefore, even if descent could be traced far back, we would have descent lines only for existing and attested languages, which would give a distorted picture of early language. As will be discussed below, at regional and even continental
scales, the languages of large areas tend to bear a certain areal resemblance to one another, and this means that some of the potential structural diversity of the world's languages has been lost to us, ironed out by pressure toward areal conformity. Some of
the world's continents show evidence of bottlenecks and founder effects in their linguistic populations,[3] and this tells us that the accidental survival and proliferation of
one language, and the accidental loss of another, can snowball into a large-scale effect
on statistical frequencies of types of languages over the course of millennia. For all of
these reasons, tracing the world's *existing* languages back to their source — even if it
were possible — would not give us an accurate picture, either genetic or structural, of
the languages spoken by the earliest humans. In view of these problems, different
means of comparison that bypass descent entirely have begun to take shape in the last
two decades. This paper summarizes some of their findings.

Family Trees

Languages fall into families, families are branches of older families, and so on.
Henceforth the oldest descent groups that can be securely demonstrated and to which

classic comparative-historical methods can be applied to yield a reconstructed protolanguage and a family tree will be called *stocks*. A stock, then, is a maximal demonstrable clade or descent group, and as mentioned above the oldest stocks average
about 6000 years old. The generic term *family* will refer here to descent groups of all
ages and all kinds (including stocks, their branches, and subbranches).

Figure 1 shows examples of some family trees, illustrated for most of the stocks of
northern Eurasia. They are schematic, showing major branches but not individual
languages. They show only branches that have survived to the present; this simplifies
the known history of Indo-European, which has early written records, so as to make it
comparable to the majority of language families that have little or no written history
and are known only from their extant daughter languages. In all the diagrams the ancestor is at the top and the descendants (daughter branches or daughter languages) at
the bottom. They are drawn to a uniform time scale, so that each is traced back for the
approximately 6000 years that linguistic science can trace descent. Consider the first
tree, that of Indo-European. Proto-Indo-European broke up and began to disperse
about 5500–6000 years ago, so in the diagram the ancestral point (or root of the tree)
and the initial branching are at the very top. Proto-Indo-European broke over the
course of about a millennium, into a large number of daughter branches, of which
eight survive (Celtic, Romance or Italic, Greek, Albanian, Armenian, Germanic,
Balto-Slavic, Indo-Iranian; extinct early branches include Tocharian of Central Asia
and the Anatolian branch which included Hittite). The daughter branches continued
to differentiate, some rather elaborately, but the diagram does not show these lower
branchings. Another family that broke up about 6000 years ago is Uralic, whose modern descendants include Hungarian, Finnish, Estonian, and the Samoyedic languages
of western Siberia. Unlike Indo-European, Uralic underwent a modest initial binary

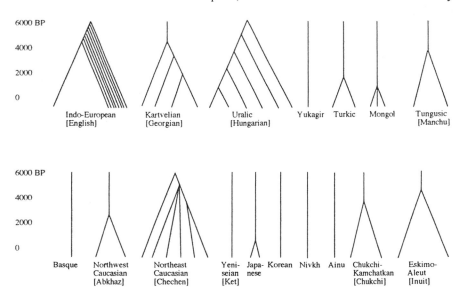

FIGURE 1. Family trees for the linguistic stocks of northern Eurasia to a constant scale, with approximate
internal branching structure corresponding to major branchings over the last *ca.* 6000 years. An example
language is named in brackets for each nonisolate stock. Only surviving stocks and branches are shown.
Major branches are shown, but not their further subdivisions. Lower parts of trees in particular are highly
schematic.

split and the subsequent history of most branches is occasional binary splits. Another stock with an initial split at about 6000 years ago is Nakh-Daghestanian (Northeast Caucasian), which underwent an initial binary split followed by more elaboration of the eastern branch.

Most of the trees have much less high-level structure. Kartvelian, whose descendants include Georgian, underwent its first split some 4000 to 4500 years ago, so the first millennium or two of its traceable existence was as a single language, shown as a straight vertical line. Similar structures with relatively late branching are found in Chukchi-Kamchatkan, Eskimo-Aleut, and Abkhaz-Circassian (Northwest Caucasian). An extreme version of this kind of history is the family tree of Basque or Yukagir or Nivkh or Ainu, in which there is no branching at all until the quite recent development of some dialect differentiation and the family tree is simply a straight line for most of the history. (Again, the diagrams show only surviving branches; extinct sisters are attested for Basque and Ket, and presumably all family trees without branching are the result of extinction of all but one daughter.) For a language like Zuni, with no significant dialectal divergence, the family tree *is* a straight line. Languages with no branching, or only recent dialect branching, in their family trees are known as *isolates*. For both isolates and families with only a few millennia of branching history, the fact that there are no demonstrable outside kin justifies extending the descent line back 6000 years, the assumption being that if there are demonstrable kin, the larger grouping is a stock and of approximately typical stock-like age, and if there are no demonstrable kin, then we know the structure of the family tree up to at least the typical stock lifespan. Isolates and small families with shallow branching dominate Figure 1, and this is the situation worldwide: Fully one-third to one-half of the world's language stocks are isolates or near-isolate shallow families. (Again, isolate status is presumably caused by extinction of sisters rather than by failure to proliferate; if actual rather than surviving branches could be shown, the diagrams in Figure 1 would probably all be extremely bushy.)

For some of these stocks, deeper connections are sometimes posited. Indo-European and Uralic are thought by many to be related, and Turkic, Mongol, and Tungusic are widely believed to be related. Proof, however, has not been offered, whereas for true stocks the genetic connection can be proved. As nonlinguists are generally not familiar with the criteria for proving that a set of languages form a family, it may be helpful to review them here. There are two kinds of criteria: genetic markers and threshold frequencies of strongly resemblant words in a carefully controlled lexical list. Both kinds of criteria rest on sufficient frequency of sufficiently close resemblances within a consistently defined grammatical or lexical set of items.

Genetic Markers

A good genetic marker is any structural feature that more or less single-handedly suffices to prove genetic relatedness. Essentially, a genetic marker is a feature or set of features whose chances of independent occurrence are so infinitesimal, and whose likelihood of diffusion is so low, that if the feature is found to recur in more than one language the most parsimonious explanation is that it is inherited from a common ancestor. Figure 2 shows the approximate pre-1600 distribution of the widespread Algonquian language family, which extends from the high plains to most of the eastern seaboard. The first native American language family encountered by English colonists, it contributed to American English a good number of words such as *skunk,*

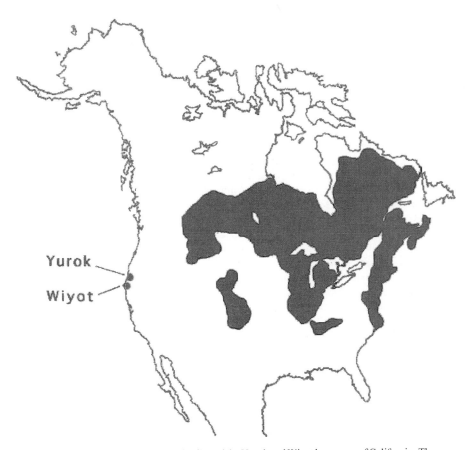

FIGURE 2. The range of the Algonquian family and the Yurok and Wiyot languages of California. The pro - nominal prefixes that prove their relatedness are:

	Proto-Algonguian	Wiyot I	II	Yurok
1st person	*ne-	du(ʔ)-	d-<*n-	ʔne-
2nd	*ke	khu(ʔ)-	kh-	k'e-
3rd	*we-	u(ʔ)-	w-	ʔwe- ≈ ʔu-

moose, sachem, wigwam, moccasin, and place names such as Manhattan, Massachu-setts, Connecticut, Passamaquoddy, Winnepesaukee, Punxsutawney, and Chicago. The foundations of an Algonquianist descriptive and comparative-historical tradition had been laid when Sapir (1913) proposed that the Algonquian family was distantly related, as one branch of a tree, to two languages of coastal northern California, Yurok and Wiyot. Given the vast jumble of languages and language families along the American Pacific coast (to be discussed below), the claim to have unearthed exactly two languages related to Algonquian was like finding two needles in a haystack. But Sapir's find was later confirmed by Haas (1958) and the theoretical groundwork of the discovery expounded by Goddard (1975). Also shown on Figure 2 is the evidence that made it possible to detect unerringly, and in short order, the relatedness of Yurok,

Wiyot, and the Algonquian family, which make up what is now known as the Algic stock: The personal pronominal prefixes. (Yurok and Wiyot, incidentally, are not close sisters. They may each be independent branches of Algic, on a par with the Algonquian family, or they may have had a period of common existence followed by a long period of independent existence.)

The pronominal prefix paradigm is the person agreement system for verbs and possessed nouns. The categories are first person ('I, me, my'), second ('you, your'), third ('he, she, it; him, her; his, her, its'), and indefinite ('someone; someone's'), and the distinctive elements are the four different initial consonants *n-, *k-, *w-, and *m-. This four-member paradigm suffices to establish genetic relatedness among the languages exhibiting it, as seems to have been realized by Sapir and Haas in their demonstration of Algic linguistic unity and as is firmly realized now and noted in all commentary on the case. (The history of the question and the definitive explanation of method are given in Goddard 1975; as noted there, the Yurok 1sg *d-* and indefinite *b-* can be shown by internal reconstruction to descend from *$*n$- and $*m$- respectively.) The statistical grounds for regarding a four-consonant paradigm as diagnostic of genetic relatedness are explained in Nichols (1996, submitted). Briefly, the logic is as follows. There are some 6000 languages on Earth; hence in a random draw any one language has a one-in-six-thousand chance of turning up. Hence 1/6000, or anything on the order of 1/10,000 (or 0.0001), represents the probability of occurrence of any random language. A secure conventional threshold of statistical significance is 0.01, and the random language's probability can be multiplied by this to yield 0.000001, or one in a million, a probability threshold which represents the likelihood of any *particular* language turning up and can be taken as a statistical definition of the unique individual language. In practical terms, this means that a linguistic subsystem with the tiny one-in-a-million or less chance of occurrence is something so unlikely to recur randomly that all tokens of such a system can confidently be assumed to descend from a single unique ancestor.

The four-consonant system of Algic pronominals meets this threshold. Since the world average for consonant phonemes is about 25 (this figure is based on my 220-language worldwide sample), any given consonant has 0.04 (1/25) chance of occurrence in any particular position in a randomly chosen word or form. The Algic pronominal system is a closed four-member opposition of person categories, and any one of the person categories has a 1/4 or 0.25 chance of occurrence in any position in the system. The Algic system with exactly those four consonants in exactly those four person categories (the full system of consonants in the respective paradigm positions attested in its entirety in each of the Algic branches) has an overall probability of 0.04 × 0.04 × 0.04 × 0.04 × 0.25 × 0.25 × 0.25 × 0.25 = 0.00000001 or one-in-a-hundred million.

For this kind of computation it is important that the various categories be strictly defined. If the consonants are defined generically (for instance, if instead of requiring specifically *n* the comparison can use any voiced dental, or if instead of specifically *k* it can use any velar obstruent, *etc.*; the ranges of variation must be set up in advance), the probability increases somewhat (a generic consonant has 0.07 probability of occurrence), though not enough to vitiate the Algic comparison.[4] What is essential is that the four person categories constitute a strict paradigm or subparadigm in each of the language families, that they occur in a fixed order with respect to the four consonant markers, and that the full system be attested in its entirety. Section (1) below shows some hypothetical pronominal systems which could be compared to the Algic one, some of which match well and indicate that the languages in question are daughters or sisters of Algic, and some of which do not match. Language (a) has the identical system suffixed rather than prefixed, and language (b) has generic consonantal resemblances; both of these languages qualify as probable Algic kin. Languages (c) and (d) have the same four consonants but (partly or entirely) in different functions. Language (e) has three of the consonants in partly different functions and a different marker for one of the functions (the cross-linguistically very common zero marking of third person). Language (f) has two of the Algic consonants in the same two functions, but different markers for the other two; in this language, the Algic paradigm is attested only partially. Language (g) has a singular/plural opposition in the person categories, and the Algic markers are randomly distributed between singular and plural. None of the non-qualifying languages are demonstrably Algic, but (f) and (g), with their first person n and second person k, are sufficiently suggestive of relatedness that a comparativist would take a second look at those languages in search of firmer evidence.

(1) The Algic pronominal system and some qualifying and nonqualifying matches to it. (a), (b), *etc.*: different languages. Sg.= singular, Pl.= plural.

	Algic	Qualifying		Nonqualifying					
		(a)	(b)	(c)	(d)	(e)	(f)	(g)	
								Sg.	Pl.
1st	n-	-n	d-	m-	k-	n-	n-	n-	sh-
2nd	k-	-k	g-	w-	n-	m-	k-	a-	k-
3rd	w-	-w	v-	k-	w-	Ø-	i-	Ø-	w-
Indef.	m-	-m	b-	n-	m-	k-	s-	m-	--

Sections (2)-(4) below show further examples of subparadigms or small paradigms that meet the threshold and suffice to demonstrate genetic relatedness. Sections (2)-(3) are from language families whose relatedness is amply evident. Both have generic resemblances of consonants and vowels. Section (4) was used by Greenberg (1960) to demonstrate genetic relatedness of Afroasiatic, the world's oldest proven genetic grouping. Greenberg's demonstration explicitly used the paradigm as sufficient evidence of relatedness, and I believe it was the first time that a genetic marker was explicitly used as sole evidence in an argument for genetic relatedness.[5]

(2) Partly suppletive third person forms of 'be' in Indo-European.

	3sg	3pl
Gothic	is	sind
Latin	est	sunt
Slavic	jestu	sõtu (*i.e.,* *soNtu) (u = short *u*; N = generic nasal)
Sanskrit	ásti	sánti
Hittite	eszi	asanzi (*i.e.,* *esti, *asanti)

(3) Germanic suppletive adjective 'good.'

	positive	comparative
English	good	better
German	gut	besser
Norwegian	god	bedre
Gothic	goths	batiza

(4) Gender-number suffixes in Afroasiatic determiners (following Greenberg 1960).

	Sing.	Pl.
Masc.	-n	
		} -n
Fem.	-t	

Shared cognates, or lexical matches more generally, can be useful as genetic markers provided the resemblances are close enough in both phonology and meaning, numerous enough in a standard wordlist, and represented frequently enough in the set of languages under comparison. Rates of vocabulary loss and threshold frequencies were discussed above. Tests using frequencies of lexical sharings to demonstrate genetic relatedness have been designed by Ringe (1992 and later works; some fine-tuning of the mathematics is in progress), Oswalt (1991), and Bender (1969). A text-book presentation of Oswalt's test is given in Trask (1996:368, 372).

Stock Density

Recall that there are some 300 linguistic stocks on Earth, a figure which is still being refined as undescribed languages receive description, and which may eventually be reduced to around 200 older lineages, but which is unlikely to be further reducible. Classificatory methodology and the genetic classification of most of the world's languages are among the great accomplishments of scientific linguistics, and the next sections of this paper show that the genetic classification can be applied to solving nongenealogical problems as well. The world's stocks, since they are genetically discrete up to the time depth of the fade-out point, provide a ready-made worldwide linguistic sample for comparative work of all kinds. The work reported here samples stocks by taking one well-described language from each major (or initial) branch of each stock. (For isolates and near-isolate shallow families, of course, there *is* only one branch.) Such a sample should contain some 400 to 500 languages, but so far mine has only 220, partly because data gathering is not complete but mostly because there are many stocks for which not even one daughter language has a satisfactory published description. Figure 3 shows the sample in its current state.

Figure 3 is also a map of genetic diversity of languages (as it was in precolonial times, in that only indigenous languages, including some now extinct, are used in the

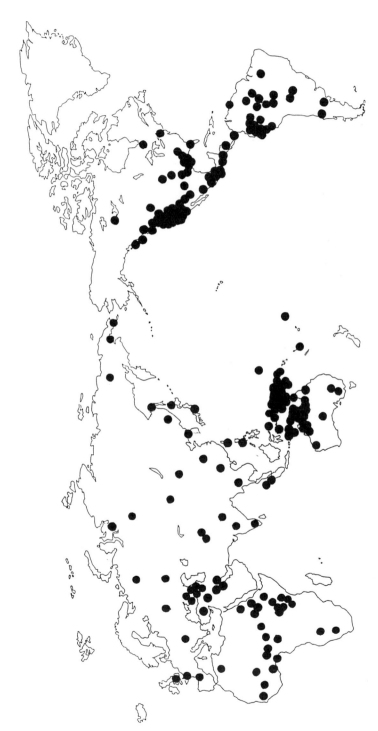

FIGURE 3. Stock-based genetic sample of the world's languages (in progress). The sample seeks one well-described language from each initial branch of each stock. South America and New Guinea are considerably undersampled. Especially in areas of high density, the plot symbol is often larger than the language's territory at map scale, and therefore the densest clusters are shown somewhat expanded. ● One sample language (approximate center of its range)

sample for the Americas, the Pacific, and Siberia). As the map shows, genetic diversity is not evenly distributed over the Earth: Linguistic stocks are densely bunched up in some areas and much more sparsely spread out in others. (This uneven distribution, incidentally, would be equally visible regardless of whether it was languages, shallow families like Romance or Slavic or Algonquian, deep families like Oceanic or Mayan or Iranian, or stocks that were sampled.) The reasons for the unevenness have been established in broad general terms (Austerlitz 1980; Birdsell 1953; Nichols 1990; Mace & Pagel 1995; Nichols 1997a): Density is favored by tropical latitude, parklike and savannah vegetation, mild and nonarid climate, low population density, and simple social structure; it is disfavored by high latitude, continuous forest, grassland or desert, arid or highly seasonal climate, high population density, and complex social structure, especially state or empire. *Stock density* is the ratio of language stocks to square miles (or kilometers) of land (this metric was proposed by Austerlitz 1980). As will be discussed again below, wherever stock density is sparse, this is the consequence of the *spread* of one or a few languages or families. Note that there are no properly linguistic factors that account for stock density; just as there is nothing in the linguistic type or structure of particular languages that leads them to develop into either elaborate or minimal family trees, so likewise there is nothing in the type or structure of languages that causes them to either bunch up or spread out.

The Age of Human Language

The first benefit of an exhaustive classification of the world's languages into strict stocks is the possibility of computing the age of human language. Recall from Figure 1 that linguistic stocks have different shapes due to different rates and extents of proliferation, and from the discussion of Figure 3 that a rapid or slow rate of proliferation is not a linguistic matter and not inborn in a language family but caused by geographic and economic factors. Let us now consider what I will call *initial branching* of language stocks: the number of distinct branches at the very top of the tree or close to it (when the tree is extended back to the approximately 6000-year limit of reconstructability). Indo-European has ten known initial branches, all of which had diverged within about a thousand years of the initial dispersal.[6] This history, however, is quite unusual. Several stocks separate initially into two branches (*e.g.*, Uralic and Northeast Caucasian in Figure 1), and the majority are either isolates (which have no branching) or shallow families (which have only a single branch for the first few millennia of their traceable lives). This same situation obtains worldwide. Several years ago I surveyed all the language stocks of the Northern Hemisphere (for which comparative work has been most thoroughly and consistently done) and found that the average number of initial branches ranges from 1.4 to 1.6. [The exact figure depends on how certain questions of language classification are resolved, and on whether Indo-European is included. The multiple initial branching of Indo-European is so unusual that excluding it from the sample drives the average down appreciably. This survey is described in Nichols (1990).]

Let us use the figure of 1.5 as the average number of initial branches of stocks. This figure, together with the approximately 6000-year age of stocks, makes it possible to compute rates of linguistic divergence and, from that, estimate the age of a group of stocks which are assumed (even if only hypothetically) to descend from a single ancestor. This is done by dividing the number of stocks by 1.5, dividing the result by 1.5, and so on until the result is less than 2; then counting the number of divisions performed and multiplying by 6000. This represents the number of stock life spans it takes to get back to approximately one ancestral stock. Table 1 shows two hypothetical applications of this procedure, and Table 2 shows the ages it gives for various numbers of stocks.

This kind of calculation is very rough (because the branching rates and stock lifespan are estimates, and because ages are even multiples of 6000) but useful. It gives a way of estimating dates of first settlement of areas, and those in turn can be used to raise hypotheses about the actual linguistic histories of areas. Some figures are shown in Table 3. (Criteria for determining the number of stocks in each area are discussed in Nichols 1997a; for Africa and northern Eurasia the higher figures are conservative counts of stocks as defined above, and the lower figures are less conservative because they count some plausible but unproven older-than-stock groupings. A full listing of the world's stocks and their representative languages in my sample will be available in a website now under design.) Consider Africa, where modern humanity probably arose some 100,000 years ago: The age of the African linguistic population, had it diverged from a single ancestor, would be at most about 42,000 years. Now, the African languages are not thought to all diverge from a single ancestor unique to them; though quite possibly some of the African stocks form one or more deep groupings, they are

Table 1. Computing the age of a set of linguistic stocks. The average stock has 1.5 initial branches. Assuming a stock age of 6000 years, divide the number of stocks by 1.5 (the average number of initial branches per stock) and repeat until the result is less than 2. Count the number of steps and multiply by 6000. (Decimals rounded to two places.) The result is the time it would take to derive this many stocks from a single ancestor (*if* they share a single ancestor, which the calculation does not establish).

		Number of stocks in the set:	
		12	30
Step:	1	$12 \div 1.5 = 8$	$30 \div 1.5 = 20$
	2	$8 \div 1.5$	$20 \div 1.5$
	3	$5.33 \div 1.5$	$13.33 \div 1.5$
	4	$3.56 \div 1.5$	$8.89 \div 1.5$
	5	$2.37 \div 1.5$	$5.93 \div 1.5$
	6		$3.95 \div 1.5$
	7		$2.63 \div 1.5$
Age:		$5 \times 6000 = 30,000$	$7 \times 6000 = 42,000$

Table 2. Estimated ages for various numbers of stocks. Calculations as in Table 1.

Number stocks	Age in years	Number stocks	Age in years
2	6000	40	48,000
3-4	12,000	60	54,000
5-6	18,000	80	60,000
7-10	24,000	100	60,000
12-15	30,000	200	72,000
20	36,000	300	78,000

ings, they are not all to be subsumed under anything younger than the ancestor of all human languages. That is, the age of the African linguistic population can be presumed on archeological grounds to be at least 100,000 years, while the age computed from the stock divergence half-life is 42,000 years. The great discrepancy between the linguistic and archeological ages of Africa indicates that there has been much extinction of linguistic diversity there, and/or loss by emigration. The same is true of northern Eurasia, which (at least at its southern periphery) has been inhabited by anatomically modern humans nearly as long as Africa, but where the linguistic age is even less than for Africa. For both of these continents the geography — high ratio of interior to coast, much of the interior either arid (Africa) or continental and seasonally cold (Eurasia) — disfavors stock diversity (cf. again Figure 3), and there has been much extinction as a result of the language spreads favored by this geography.

A somewhat similar picture obtains for Australia, where the number of indigenous language stocks yields a linguistic age less than the archeological age. (For early dates in Australia see Roberts et al. 1990, Roberts & Jones 1994.) On the other hand, the linguistic age of New Guinea, and of Australia-New Guinea together, is 60,000 years, close to the archeological date of 50,000+ years. (Australia and New Guinea were a single landmass during the last glaciation, when water was locked up in glaciers and sea levels were low, exposing the continental shelf. Hence their early human settlement history is shared.) That Australia has a distinctly younger linguistic age than New Guinea is a consequence of Australia's geography with its sizable arid interior which fosters language spreads and extinctions. Still, even for New Guinea the linguistic age is misleading: Multiple colonization is known to have occurred, probably from the very beginning (see e.g., White 1996; Nichols 1997b), hence the languages cannot be presumed to have descended from a single unique ancestor. If the modern linguistic diversity is what would have descended from only one initial colonization, then even here some extinction has evidently taken place.

The case of the Americas is different. Here the linguistic age is much greater than the archeological age. As will be discussed below, the discrepancy is due in part to multiple colonization, but even when that is factored in the linguistic age is greater than the known archeological age.

Thus comparing linguistic and archeological ages of continents can be informative in various ways, but it cannot straightforwardly indicate actual colonization dates; linguistic dates are most useful when they are either much younger than archeological dates and therefore give clear evidence of extinction of linguistic lines (as in Africa) or much older than archeological dates, thereby indicating multiple colonization (as in the Americas).

This much holds for linguistic ages of continent-sized populations of languages, where dates of first colonization and frequency of colonizations complicate the picture. But what of the age of human language in general? Table 3 shows that the linguistic age of the entire world population of linguistic stocks is only 72,000 to 78,000 years — much too young, given that modern language is probably at least as old as anatomically modern humanity. Here, as with Africa, the discrepancy is due to patterns of extinction. A more accurate estimate of the world's linguistic age is shown in the last two entries in Table 3, where the number of stocks is the number that would be expected if the entire traditionally inhabited world were populated with language stocks at the density attested in the Americas or — most accurately — New Guinea, which has the world's highest stock density.[7] The outcome is that to populate the traditionally inhabited world with language families at the density that can be reached when circumstances are favorable — that of New Guinea — would take some

Table 3. Estimated ages for some actual linguistic populations. Calculations as in Ta ble 1. Descent of each population from a single ancestor is assumed for the calculation, but is not supported by linguistic evidence or (with the possible exception of the entire world) generally believed by linguists. Ar chaeological age is the oldest generally accepted dated site or human remains; as the criteria are conservative and older sites may exist but not have been found, archaeological age is a minimum age of habitation.

Area	Number stocks	Linguistic Age in Ky	Archaeological age in Ky
Africa (low)	17	36	100
Africa (high)	30	42	100
Northern Eurasia	16-18	36	90?
New Guinea	80	60	50+
Australia	20?	36	50+
New Guinea and Australia	100	60	50+
North America	50	48	13
North and Central America	60	54	13
Entire World	≈130	66	13
World (low)	200	72	
World (high)	300	78	
World at New World density	466	84	
World at New Guinea density	≈12,000	132	

132,000 years. This is then the linguistic age of the world. If the world's language stocks descend from a single ancestor, then that ancestor began to diversify at least 132,000 years ago.[8] This computation does not tell us whether the world's languages descend from a single ultimate ancestor. But if they do, then that ancestor language began to disperse well before the anatomically modern physical type began to spread.

Ages for Some Possible Ancient Lineages

Although the maximum age for demonstrated stocks is about 6000 years, there are a few groupings of stocks that are widely regarded as probable sisters whose genetic unity is too ancient to be amenable to standard reconstruction. The clearest example is Afroasiatic, a group of African stocks whose genetic unity is proved by several different genetic markers (see Greenberg 1960, 1963; Newman 1980) but for which regular correspondences and reconstruction cannot be demonstrated to the satisfaction of the field. [Two recent comprehensive proposals for correspondences and reconstructions are Orel & Stolbova (1995) and Ehret (1995), but neither has won general acceptance.] The surviving branches of Afroasiatic number from four to seven depending on how questions of subgrouping are resolved: Berber, whose internal differentiation is very recent; Chadic, an old family; Semitic, a very old family of stock-like age; Cushitic, now often divided into two or three stock-like branches (northern Cushitic, southern Cushitic, and isolate Beja); and probably Omotic. (Ancient Egyptian and its descendant Coptic represent another branch of Afroasiatic which, however, has not survived and therefore does not figure in the age computation.) Various proposals unite Berber with one more branches (Chadic, Semitic, Cushitic) (proposals and overviews of Afroasiatic include Bender 1975, 1997;Diakonoff 1988; Newman 1980; Greenberg 1963).

By the half-life computation, depending on the branching structure assumed, the age of Afroasiatic is from 12,000 years for four branches to 24,000 years for seven. The calculation assumes that Afroasiatic has a normal branching rate and a typical higher-level branching structure (though of course it cannot identify the actual branches and propose a specific subgrouping): If there are seven stock-level branches now, 6000 years ago there were 4.67, *i.e.*, under five, and 12,000 years ago there were 3.11, *i.e.*, about three; if there are four branches now, 6000 years ago there were 2.67 and 12,000 years ago there were 1.78, *i.e.*, under two. Because the calculation can only measure age in 6000-year increments, any adjustment in branching structure (such as division of Cushitic or union of Berber with another branch) has a drastic effect on the computed age for a relatively small set of stocks like this one. Thus the results of linguistic comparative reconstruction bear heavily on the computable age of Afroasiatic. Positing fewer subgroups that unite more stocks lowers the age; positing numerous binary splits raises the age. Uniting any of the branches into true stocks will lower the age. The strongest case for a great age for Afroasiatic would come from a demonstration that it has a complex hierarchical internal branching structure; this would show that the computation of a regular half-life is plausible.

This discussion of Afroasiatic shows that the half-life with its large increments is a very crude measure of age for relatively recent events, but that combined with close comparative work on branching substructure its accuracy can be improved. In addition, note that even with questions of higher branching structure unresolved it is clear that the age of Afroasiatic is likely to be closer to 12,000 years than to 6000, and perhaps over 12,000. This is by far the oldest securely demonstrated linguistic lineage on Earth. (Recall, however, that Afroasiatic has so far eluded reconstruction, that there is much debate about its higher-level branching structure, and that it is by far the clearest case of an older-than-stock grouping. These considerations justify using 6000 years as the best estimate of the average fade-out point.) Some proposed but unproven groupings of comparable age are discussed below.

Monogenesis of Language?

Do the world's languages in fact ultimately descend from a single ancestor, a Proto-World as it is often called? Or were there several ancestral languages? The latter situation — polygenesis — would have obtained if premodern language evolved into modern language separately more than once in more than one distinct population, or if the evolution of modern language took place gradually in a human population large enough to consist of several different language communities. These are two very different scenarios: The first implies that the evolutionary process occurred more than once, each time in a single speech community, while the second implies that the evolutionary process occurred only once, but affected a population of several speech communities simultaneously. Monogenesis — one-time-only development of modern language out of just one ancestral premodern language — implies either a unique gradual evolution of just one premodern language into a modern language, or sudden appearance of modern language in one individual or household or clan with a sharp discontinuity from whatever preceded and from whatever was in use next door.

These are very different scenarios: The first involves a unique occurrence of a common sort of gradual evolutionary change, while the second implies a fairly drastic saltatory change. Thus we have, in all, four possible scenarios. The two polygenetic scenarios both imply multiple ancestors to modern languages, and the two monogenetic scenarios both imply a single ancestor.

There is of course no way of establishing the number of ultimate ancestral languages by tracing descent, but a rough estimate of the number — or at least a well-founded conjecture as to whether the ancestors were one or many — can be derived from linguistic geography and the study of contact-induced language change. Tropical foraging societies tend to be small in favorable geographical and climatic conditions, averaging at most about 500 individuals in what I will call the *ethnolinguistic unit*, the tribe-like group speaking a single language. (For the figure of 500 see Birdsell 1953; for comparison linguistic figures see Nichols 1990. The smallest groups are found where cultures are simplest, population density is thin, and the environment is tropical and nonarid, factors that obtained for early humans.) Therefore, an estimate of the total population size for earliest *Homo sapiens* will make it possible to estimate an approximate number of small to average-sized ethnolinguistic units. The following argument is something of a thought experiment using this and other plausible assumptions about paleosociolinguistics.

Though I know of no precise figures on the matter, in a society as small as 500 individuals some intermarriage with neighboring ethnolinguistic units is likely, especially if there are large-scale internal exogamous groupings such as clans, sections, or moieties that restrict one's choice of marriage partners beyond the usual close kinship constraints. In all cases that I am aware of where ethnolinguistic groups are very small, intermarriage with neighboring groups is common, even systematic. Intermarriage often means bilingualism — fairly uniform society-wide bilingualism if there are standing intermarriage patterns between two societies, and more diverse household-by-household bilingualism or multilingualism where intermarriage patterns involve more societies and are more varied. Now, systematic and long-term bilingualism or multilingualism can entail convergence between the languages involved (for convergence see Thomason & Kaufman 1988; case studies of multilingualism in small societies include Ross 1996; Heath 1978). Thus, from small group size we can infer likely bilingualism and multilingualism, and from that we can infer likely convergence at least among neighboring languages and perhaps over the entire early human range, depending on its size and layout.

There are several different hypotheses about the population size, location, and territorial range of the ancestral modern humans. On the one most widely held, modern humans emerged over 100,000 years ago in the riverine and lacustrine environment of eastern Africa, spreading into the Old World tropics and eastern Mediterranean area sometime thereafter, perhaps around 80,000 years ago and certainly by 50,000 years ago.[9] Let us now combine this scenario with what is known about linguistic geography and language contact. The range within which our ancestors evolved was roughly linear, somewhat over 2000 miles long and a few hundred miles wide (from the vicinity of Lake Turkana down the Rift Valley and continuing to southernmost Africa). These are dimensions comparable to New Guinea, which harbors great diversity of language families and has some distinct internal linguistic subareas as well as a certain amount of overall areality in features which spread easily, such as word order and sound systems.

There is good reason to believe that modern language evolved gradually within a sizable population, rather than abruptly in a small advanced social circle. The modern brain and speech apparatus appear to have evolved slowly, gradually, and relatively uniformly over the entire species. Modern language depends for its proper transmission on both the inherited language faculty and proper exposure at the right age, and the set of inherited apparatus, inherited learning capacity, and actual learning could not arise spontaneously and abruptly. In addition, abrupt appearance of full-blown modern language in one individual or family in a society speaking a more primitive form of language would have been an evolutionary saltation that would have fractured the society and compromised its viability. For all of these reasons it is safe to assume that at no time during the long and gradual emergence of modern language were there marked differences within the species as to the degree of modernity of language.

Estimates of the size of the earliest modern human population at about 100,000 years ago range from a few tens of thousands to a million or more.[10] Even the smallest of these figures would allow for a good number of distinct ethnolinguistic groups, and the territorial range over which early modern humans are found virtually guarantees considerable linguistic diversity. The closest historically attested analogs to this combination of low population density, riverine-lacustrine environment with savannah interface, tropical climate, and foraging economy are probably northern Australia and (albeit horticultural) lowland New Guinea and parts of northern South America. These areas all accommodate considerable numbers of language families.

On the other hand, the probable small size of the early ethnolinguistic groups suggests intermarriage and multilingualism and hence convergence at least locally; here, too, the analogs I am familiar with (Australia, New Guinea) are marked by a good deal of multilingualism and some degree of local to regional linguistic convergence. As the range was more or less linear, convergence patterns would have been chainlike, with the languages at the far northern and southern ends of the chain greatly distinct from each other in structure as well as descent.[11]

Taking into account all of the factors discussed here, it is likely that the human linguistic population prior to the expansion out of Africa consisted of perhaps a hundred distinct languages falling into perhaps ten distinct stock-like genetic lineages and showing several distinct areal patterns of typological resemblance and probably a good deal of typological diversity over the entire range.[12] To populate the traditionally inhabited world at New Guinea densities from an ancestral population of 10 stocks would require 108,000 years, a time frame reaching back to the eve of the dispersal of anatomically modern humans.

Thus modern language in its earliest existence was probably a population of languages with internal genetic and structural diversity and some local and general areality. When the spread of modern humans out of Africa began, the northern part of the ancestral linguistic range must have been a disproportionate contributor of emigrant linguistic populations, but nonetheless over the millennia the languages that spread out represented a good swath of the range of ancestral linguistic diversity, both genetic and structural.

Homo erectus appeared nearly two million years ago and soon thereafter spread over Africa and southern Europe and Asia, in all probability carrying primitive languages which continued to diversify and diverge for over a million years. Presumably Africa continued to be a center of slow biological and linguistic spread thereafter; the distinctive physiology of modern humans, following the same origin and trajectory much later, made the spread trajectory visible. Modern language, and descent lineages of languages, must have followed the same trajectory, but the spread of modern language need not have coincided exactly with the spread of modern physiology and, as argued above, may have preceded it.

Thus the east African linguistic population within which modern language evolved is likely to have been a genetic and structural subset of world linguistic diversity of its time, and this means that modern language, though polygenetic, is not maximally polygenetic: Most of the linguistic lineages of premodern humanity died out when modern humanity and modern language spread. Whether the range of modern structural diversity of languages is restricted as a result of this ancient skewing is unknown and probably unknowable. What is clear is that when modern humans spread across southern Eurasia and beyond between about 70,000 and 50,000 years ago the languages of the previous inhabitants at the periphery had been diversifying for at least the few hundred thousand years of archaic modern humans and perhaps the entire nearly two-million-year lifespan of *Homo erectus*. This was the greatest degree of genetic diversity that has ever existed in human and hominid language, and it went extinct without a trace.

The Spread of Languages Over the World

Sample and Historical Markers

This section will summarize research published in detail elsewhere (Nichols 1992, 1995a, 1997a; Nichols & Peterson 1996) and show that the relative frequencies of diagnostic structural features in large areally-based sets of languages can reveal fundamental affinities between some of these populations, and that these in turn point to shared geographical origins. This approach bypasses descent entirely and instead traces nongenealogical affinities between large geographically-based groupings of language families. It cannot trace the origins of individual families very well, but it can trace the settlement of continents, explain the worldwide geographic distribution of language families, and reach very far back into prehistory.

For purposes of interarea comparison, the sample is divided into 18 subcontinent-sized areas: Southern Africa, northern Africa, the Caucasus and the languages of ancient Mesopotamia, Europe, inner Asia, northeastern Asia (= eastern Siberia, roughly), southeast Asia, coastal New Guinea and Melanesia, interior and southern New Guinea, northern coastal Australia, southern and interior Australia, the American Pacific northwest (from Alaska to Oregon), California, the Great Basin and Plains, eastern North America, Mesoamerica, western South America, and eastern South America. These areas are defined in purely geographical terms and set up so as to contain roughly equal numbers of sample languages. Various structural features are surveyed in the sample languages, and the 18 areas are compared in terms of the relative frequencies of those features in the area's languages. The 18 sample areas are shown in Figure 4.

The database of sample languages and sampled structural features was designed in order to seek out statistically significant differences in features across areas, differences that would point to geographical origins for populations of languages much as frequencies of blood types, mitochondrial DNA lineages, *etc.*, in human populations point to geographical origins for those populations. (In both cases it is individual lineages within the population, and not the entire population as such, that have geographical origins, but reaching statistical significance requires comparing populations.) The structural features chosen for this first comparison were ones that observation had suggested were relatively persistent in language families, of relatively low frequency worldwide, not readily diffused, and not likely to arise spontane-

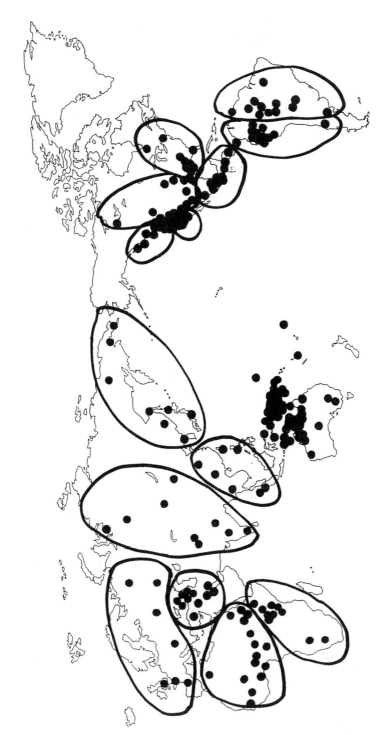

FIGURE 4. Sample languages, with the eighteen large sample areas shown.

ously. The presence of such a feature in a language or language population is likely to be due to inheritance or direct, close contact and unlikely to be due to universals, indirect or superficial contact, or accident. If a usably large set of such features can be found, statistically significant differences in their frequencies from area to area are likely to point to shared origins or shared population history. Such features can be called *historical markers,* and a long-term goal of historically-oriented comparative grammar is to amass as large as possible a set of reliable historical markers. Fortunately, the dozen or so prospective historical markers pursued in this survey have all proven useful in their cross-linguistic statistical patterning, and comparative typological work (Nichols 1992, 1995b) has shown that they are reasonably independent of each other, persistent in language families, not prone to spontaneous innovation, and reliably extractable from published grammatical descriptions.

Sections (5)-(7) below illustrate some of the historical markers used in the work reported here. (It should be cautioned that the inventory of markers is biased toward morphological ones.) Sections (5)-(6) are examples from Ingush, a language of the Northeast Caucasian family spoken in southern Russia, illustrating *ergativity,* the identical grammatical coding of subject of intransitive verb and direct object of intransitive, while the subject of a transitive verb is coded differently. In (5), the verb 'gave' is transitive; the subject *Muusaa-z* is in the ergative case, an oblique case specialized for marking subjects of transitive verbs; the direct object *axcha* 'money' is in the nominative case, the basic case or citation form, which has no suffix; and the verb agrees in gender (shown by its prefix) with the direct object. In (6) the verb is intransitive; *Muusaa* is subject and in the nominative case, and the verb agrees with it in gender. Ergativity is a low-frequency feature worldwide (only some 25% of the languages in the 220-language sample exhibit it to some degree), and Figure 5 shows that its distribution is skewed: It is very frequent in the Caucasus and Australia, fairly well attested in highland New Guinea and central Eurasia, and rare elsewhere. These differences are statistically significant, and therefore cannot be assumed to be due to random chance or language universals.

(5) Ingush   Muusaa-z   shii   voʕ-a   axcha   d-alar
            Musa (V)-ERG his   son-DAT   money (D)   D-gave
            'Musa gave his son money'
            (Case name abbreviations: ERGative, DATive; D = gender prefix;
            (V), (D) = gender of nouns.)

(6) Ingusb   Muusaa   aara - v-ealar
            Musa (V)   out   V-went
            'Musa went out'

Ingush is a dependent-marking language in which grammatical relations such as subject, object, and possessor are marked primarily by cases on the nouns and pronouns. In (7), in contrast, taken from Abkhaz of the Northwest Caucasian family (spoken in western Georgia), nouns bear no cases, the verb agrees elaborately with the subject, indirect object, and direct object, and in general heads of constituents agree with their dependents; Abkhaz is a head-marking language. Head-marking languages are not frequent worldwide, except in the Americas where they abound (Figure 6). Head marking is another historical marker.

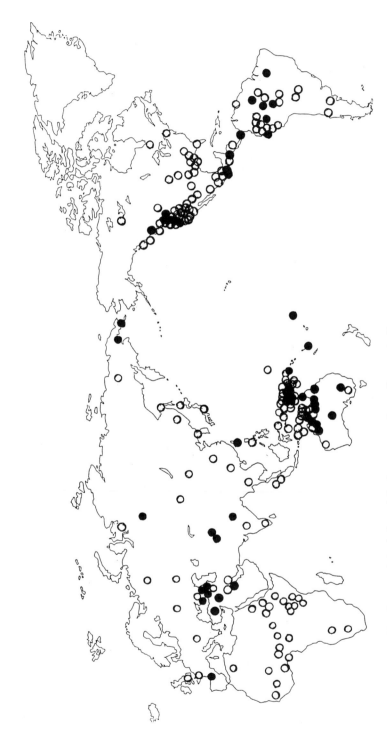

FIGURE 5. Languages with salient morphological ergativity (in noun or verb paradigms, or both).

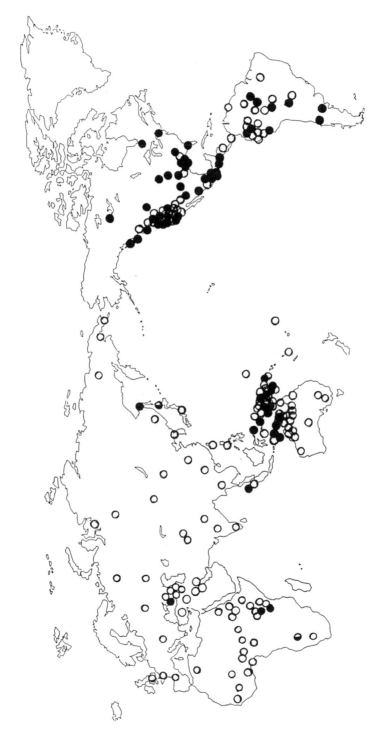

FIGURE 6. Head-marking languages. ● Head-marking languages of moderate to high morphological complexity. ◐ Head-marking languages of very low complexity. ○ Non-head-marking languages.

(7) Abkhaz   a - xaca   a - pʰ°əs   a - sq°'ə   Ø - lə - y - te - yt'
              the man   the woman   the book   it   to her   he give   PAST
              'The man gave the woman a book'

Identical stems in singular and plural forms of personal pronouns provide another historical marker. Here first person pronouns have been surveyed as the single best indicator of this tendency. Section (8) shows identical stems in two languages of California. In Yawlumni (Yawelmani Yokuts), the plural forms are derived from the singular forms by suffixation. In Wintu, there is no singular/plural distinction but only a person distinction, so it can be said that singular and plural forms are completely identical. Identical singular/plural stems are uncommon worldwide yet frequent in a few areas (Figure 7).

Section (8) also illustrates personal pronoun systems with first person *n* and second person *m*. Such systems again are rare worldwide but common along an extended stretch of Pacific coast in the Americas (Figure 8; Nichols & Peterson 1996).

(8) Personal pronouns in selected native American languages. sg. = singular, pl .= plural.

	Yawlumni		Wintu	Cashinahua	
	sg.	pl.	sg. = pl.	sg.	pl.
1st	na?	na?an	ni	en, e-	nun, nuku
2nd	ma?	ma?an	mi	min, mi-	man, matu

The rest of this section summarizes recent work that makes use of these historical markers in order to trace the spread of languages around the Pacific Rim. The modern distribution of historical markers is the only evidence we have of the ancient spread of languages from an origin probably in the vicinity of southeastern Asia to New Guinea, Australia, and Oceania on the one hand and to northern Asia, Beringia, and the New World on the other, and for the chronology of those spreads.

Only the general fact of language spread can be inferred from the distribution of the markers. Just how a language has spread — by migration of the speaker population, demographic expansion of the speaking population, shift of the speech community to the language of a prestigious or powerful neighbor, or some combination of these — cannot be inferred. Nor can it be inferred whether a given language has inherited a given historical marker or acquired it through close direct contact. All that can be assumed is that statistically significant sharing of historical markers between languages or language families points to a common geographical origin of the languages or families, and statistically significant sharing of historical markers between two or more populations points to a common geographical origin of some component of the populations. The sociolinguistics of the transmission scenario and the spreads cannot be reconstructed from the distribution of the markers, but this is no obstacle to reconstructing the abstract fact of language spread and the trajectories and chronologies of spread.

The method used here has been explicated previously (Nichols 1992: Ch. 6, 1995a, 1997b, c; Nichols & Peterson 1996). Fifteen or more historical markers are traced across the sample languages and their relative frequencies (languages showing

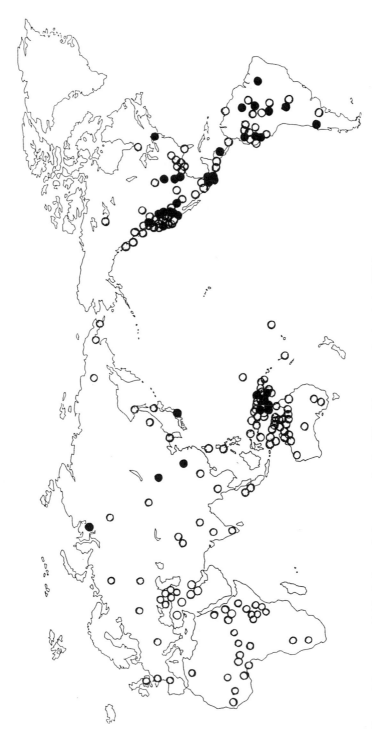

FIGURE 7. Languages with identical stems in first person singular ('1') and first person plural exclusive ('We') pronouns.

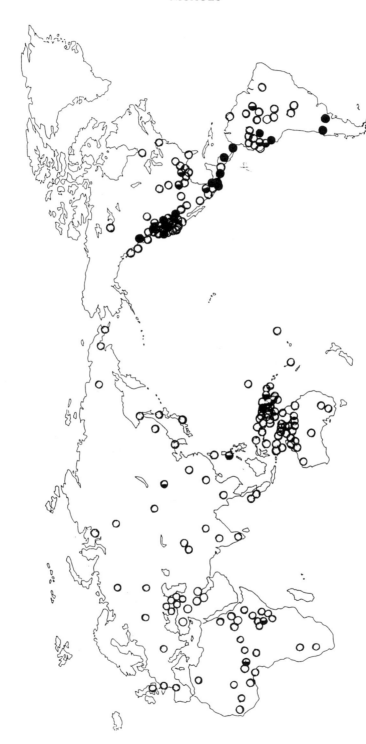

FIGURE 8. Languages with personal pronouns having *n* as first consonant in the first person singular and *m* as first consonant in the second person singular.

the feature as a percent of the languages of the area) are counted in each of the 18 large areas listed above (or some similar geographically-based breakdown of a dozen or more areas). They are also plotted on a map. Any skewings in their cross-areal frequencies that are statistically significant are taken to be non-accidental and indicators of a common origin. An origin and spread scenario are reconstructed to the extent possible by comparing the linguistic distribution to what is known of prehistory from archeological and other sources.

Worldwide Longitudinal Ranking of Areas

As tabulated in Nichols (1997c), for each of the historical markers the 18 areas were ranked by frequency of the marker in the area, then either the rank steps or the distance in steps from the first-ranked area was totaled for each of the areas.[13] The re-

TABLE 4. Sum of rankings of areas, based on frequencies of historical markers in them. Lineariz ation is schematic; a space means a relatively large distance between areas. An asterisk (*) marks ar eas that are out of place, and the notes to the right comment on this.

Europe	Europe is at the far western periphery of the world
Caucasus	
North Africa	Africa is western and peripheral
South Africa	Africa is western and peripheral
*Australian interior	Interior Australia is in the western Old World
Northeast Asian coast	
*New Guinea interior	Interior New Guinea is in the western Old World
Inner Asia	
*Australia coast	Coastal Australia is in Asia
Southeast Asia	
Eastern North America	
California	
Basin - Plains	
Western South America	
Eastern South America	
Alaska - Oregon	
*New Guinea coast	Coastal New Guinea is in western America and
Mesoamerica	(With Mesoamerica) at the far eastern periphery

sults are shown in Table 4: The relative frequencies of historical markers worldwide correspond rather well to geographical longitude, with Europe and Africa at one extreme (which can be considered the western edge) and the Americas at the other (which can be considered the eastern edge). This basically linear distribution, running from what can be called a western pole in the vicinity of Africa to an eastern pole in the Americas, is a schematic geography of the traditionally inhabited world from the initial dispersals of modern humans and modern languages up to the end of the first millennium AD, when the Viking era brought the first known transgression of the western pole and the first known colonization of the Americas from the western Old World.

Variants of this computation, using a different inventory of historical markers, different scales of areal breakdown, a somewhat different inventory of sample languages, and/or (as mentioned in Note 13) different bellwether areas for determining whether rank sorts would be ascending or descending, yield essentially the same results (the main difference between the variants is some jockeying for last place among the American subcontinents). The results are thus reasonably robust. The strongest determinant of the relative frequencies of structural features in language populations is longitude, and the cline of frequency rankings of areas is also an approximate schematic linear map of the premodern distribution of our species and our languages. The salient departures from literal geographical longitude in Table 4 — the westward displacement of Australia and interior New Guinea to western Eurasia and the eastward displacement of coastal New Guinea to the southern Americas — are discussed immediately below.

Coastal Spread Around the Pacific Rim

Based on their frequencies of historical markers, the language areas around the Pacific fall into three large groups which, although each is spread over several continents and two hemispheres, exhibit a degree of internal cohesion and external continuity that suggests a single historical origin for each of the three and a regular chronological continuity between them. I will call these larger areas *provinces*. The most clearly demarcated province can be called the Pacific Rim province, as it clusters at or near the coastline all around the Pacific. Figures 7 and 8 above, and Figure 9-12 below, show the diagnostic historical markers of the Pacific Rim province: identical singular and plural pronominal stems, $n : m$ personal pronoun roots, numeral classifiers, verb-initial word order, tones, and possessive classification.[14] These markers cluster around the Pacific coast of New Guinea (but not Australia), Asia, North America, and Southern America. Numeral classifiers, $n : m$ pronoun roots, and possessive classification are found almost exclusively around and near the Pacific Rim. Tones and verb-initial order are well represented in the western Old World, but in Asia, Australasia, and the New World they again cluster near the coast. Identical singular and plural pronoun stems and $n : m$ pronoun systems have a sparse coastally oriented distribution in Asia and Australasia but a more abundant coastally oriented distribution in the Americas, perhaps suggesting founder effects. Taken together, the five markers show continuity and an overall coastal orientation almost entirely around the Pacific Rim.

The next province can be called the Pacific Hinterland. It is not clearly distinct from the Pacific Rim province, but is marked by a few features that are common in the Rim province and also extend farther inland and to northern Australia. These features are head-marking morphology, shown in Figure 6, and gender or other agree-

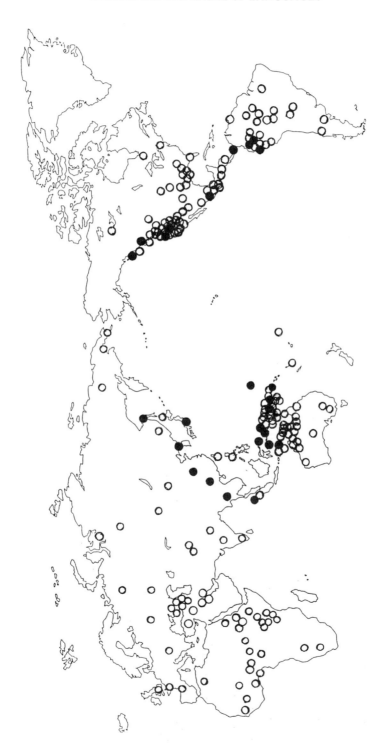

FIGURE 9. Languages having numeral classifiers.

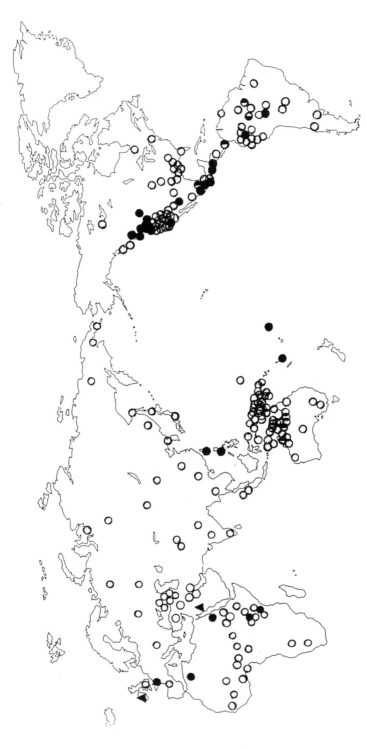

FIGURE 10. Languages with verb-initial basic word order. Schematically (V = verb, S = subject, O = direct object): ● VSO or VOS. ◑ VS but SOV or SVO. ◐ OVS. ○ VSO or VOS. ▲ Well-known languages not in sample (Irish, Arabic).

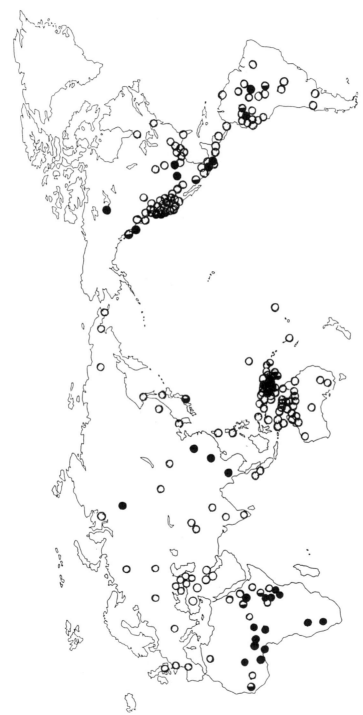

FIGURE 11. Languages with tones. ● Elaborate tone system (tones on all or most syllables of the word). ◑ Minimal systems (tones on one accented syllable only).

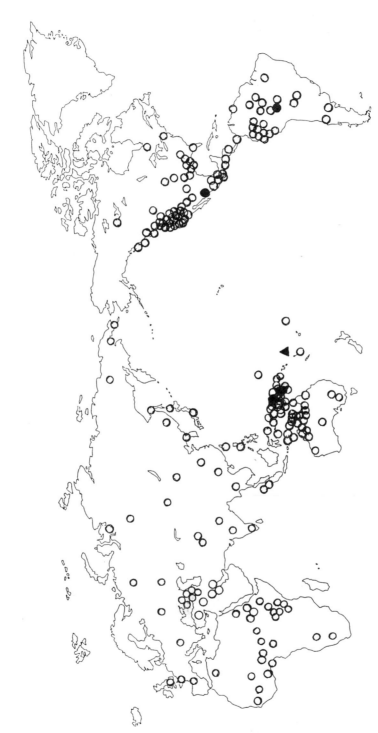

FIGURE 12. Possessive classification of nouns. Distinct inflectional classes of nouns that become evident only when possessive affixes are added. ▲ Language not in sample

ment classes in nouns, shown in Figure 13. Three other features appear to have this distribution, but they have not yet been fully surveyed: Reduplicated plurals; extensive prefixation; and causativization as a regular derivational process in the verbal lexicon.

More distinct in its linguistic properties, but more diffuse geographically, is the Pacific Interior province consisting of interior Australia, interior New Guinea, eastern South America, and to some extent eastern North America. It is distinguished by ergativity (Figure 5), rarity of head-marking morphology and frequency of dependent-marking morphology (Figure 14), systematic marking of singular/plural (or singular/dual/plural) oppositions on nouns, minimal consonant systems (often limited to a single manner of articulation), and high frequency of derived intransitivity in the verbal lexicon (these last three have not been fully surveyed and are not mapped here).

The structural affinities between interior Australia, interior New Guinea, and the eastern New World explain some of the departures from literal geographical longitude in the linear typological geography of Table 4. The interiors of Australia and New Guinea are closer to each other in Table 4 than either is to its own coast, and both are displaced far to the west, a distribution that reflects both the unity of the Interior province and the fact that many of its distinctive markers are also common in western Eurasia and in Africa. Coastal New Guinea belongs to the Pacific Rim province and is drawn far to the east in the linear map, ending up as a neighbor of the American Pacific coastal areas. The northern coast of Australia is part of the Pacific hinterland and lies well to the east of the Australian interior but well to the west of the Pacific Rim.

The maps in Figures 5–14 show that all three provinces are cut off, as it were, in the north; the Eskimo-Aleut, Chukchi-Kamchatkan, and Tungusic language families that dominate northern Siberia find most of their typological affinities to the west, among the languages of central Eurasia, and their considerable weight in the sample draws the Northeast Asian sample area somewhat to the west.

These distributions can point to geographical origins of languages and to the history of linguistic colonization around the Pacific. Some basic assumptions need to be made about Pacific colonization. The human populations that colonized the lands around the Pacific can be assumed to have emanated ultimately from eastern Asia: People moved from mainland southeast Asia through insular southeast Asia to colonize Australasia some 50,000 years ago, and from coastal and/or interior northern Asia via Beringia to colonize the Americas. (This assumption seems to be the received view in archeology and human genetics.) The linguistic populations of the colonized areas can also be presumed to derive from eastern Asia; this much can be assumed even without knowing the sociolinguistic and historical specifics of the language spreads. I also assume that any linguistic population in the right part of eastern Asia would have been positioned to see some of its descendants move northward and ultimately into the Americas and others move southward and ultimately into Australasia.

On these assumptions, the following interpretation of historical marker distributions can be given. The Interior province is dominated by descendants of a very early wave of colonization, a wave that began in some critically positioned part of eastern Asia and is now best represented in the most distant and presumably last-reached parts of very separate areas: the east, south, and interior of Australia, the interior of New Guinea, lowland and eastern South America, and to a lesser extent eastern North America. In both Australasia and the New World, this province includes a great range of climatic and geographical conditions, settlement of which required a variety of

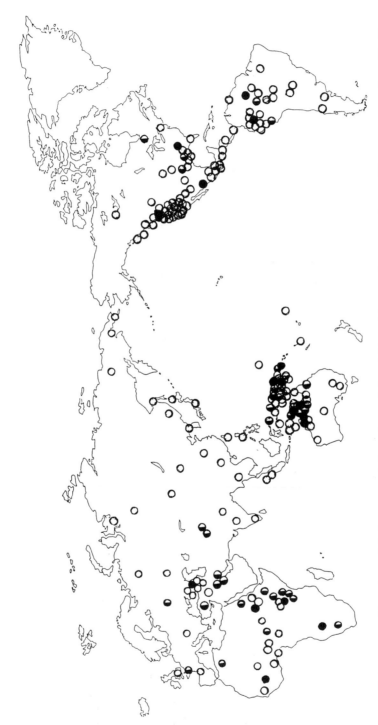

FIGURE 13. Languages with genders and similar agreement classes (concord classes). Nouns trigger gender agreement on modifiers, pronouns, verbs, and/or other words. ● Five or more genders. ◐ Two to four genders.

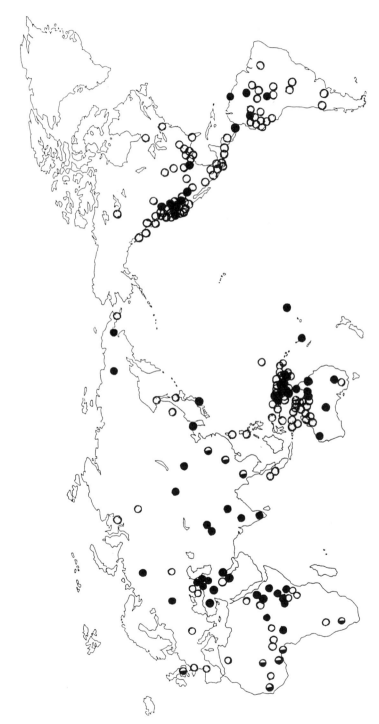

FIGURE 14. Dependent-marking languages. ● Dependent-marking languages with moderate to high morphological complexity. ◑ Dependent-marking languages with very low morphological complexity. ○ Nondependent-marking languages.

secondary adaptations on the part of the colonizers (whose entry points were the northwest coast and offshore islands of then-united Australia-New Guinea, and of Alaska). The longer the residence in the colonized area, the greater the chance of spread to the distant points and extreme environments; hence descendants of earliest immigrants are disproportionately represented in these far reaches. The movement of first-wave languages into the colonized continents probably involved a relatively high proportion of language spread by human migration, as the lands were minimally inhabited or uninhabited at first.

The Pacific Hinterland province is a slightly expanded coastally oriented area. It suggests a later colonization impulse which was coastal and retained a primarily coastal orientation throughout a sizable spread along the northern coasts of Australia and New Guinea and the entire Pacific region of North, Central, and South America. This is a more recent stratum which has not penetrated far into the interior of Australia, New Guinea, or the Americas. The Pacific Rim province is still more recent; it is more strictly coastal, geographically more restricted (not reaching Australia at all), and sharply delimited by the feature distributions on the maps in Figures 7–12. Its geography and the sharpness of its linguistic profile mark it as a recently formed area. In the case of both the Pacific Hinterland and the Pacific Rim provinces, the coastal orientation was retained perhaps because coastally adapted immigrants remained coastal and carried their languages with them, or perhaps because immigrants entered a coastal cultural and linguistic area that favored diffusion and language spread through shift.

Finally, after the Pacific Rim population had entered the Americas, Proto-Eskimo-Aleut and Proto-Chukchi-Kamchatkan entered the coastal sphere in the north and spread, cutting off the continuity of the Asian and American Pacific Rim populations and representing the first appearance of the interior Eurasian linguistic type in America (Figure 15).

The Ages of the Circum-Pacific Spreads

A reliable though approximate relative and absolute chronology can be worked out for the Pacific Rim province. On the near side it is bounded in the Americas by the spread of the Eskimo-Aleut family in the north. The Eskimo-Aleut language family lacks the historical markers of the Pacific Rim province, and its structural type is strongly reminiscent of the languages of interior Siberia and central Asia: It is ergative, suffixing, case-using, consistently distinguishes number in nouns and pronouns, and lacks tones and numeral classifiers. The family is probably some 4000 to 5000 years in age (Woodbury 1984) and almost certainly dispersed in the vicinity of southwestern Alaska where its Aleut and Eskimoan branches now meet, but linguistic sources are of the unanimous opinion that it is a relatively recent entrant to the New World from Siberia. Similar to Eskimo-Aleut in type is the Chukchi-Kamchatkan family, comparable in age to Eskimo-Aleut and indigenous to coastal Siberia, originating probably between the bases of the Chukotkan and Kamchatkan peninsulas. (For this family and a map of the Beringian languages see Krauss 1988. For historical connections of Eskimo-Aleut and Chukchi-Kamchatkan see Fortescue 1998.) Thus it appears that as of about 5000 years ago the Pacific Rim province had been separated in the north by an entering wedge of languages of interior Eurasian type, led by Eskimo-Aleut and followed by Chukchi-Kamchatkan.

In Australasia there is a clear date for the beginning of the Pacific Rim stratum (Nichols 1997b). The two earlier provinces are found in both Australia and New

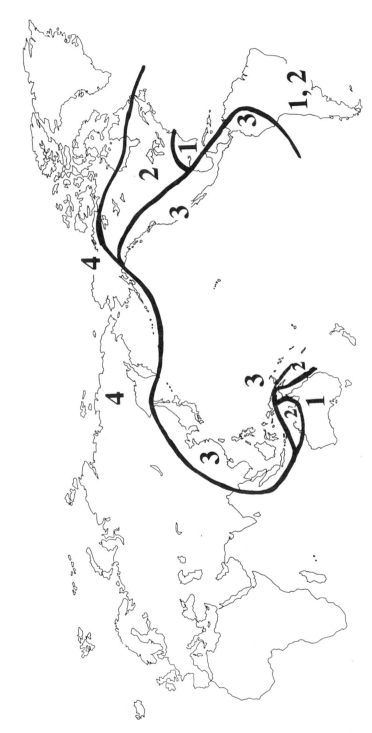

FIGURE 15. Schematic model of four waves of New World and Pacific colonization from Asia (after Nichols 1995: 214). Chronological stratification: (1) Pacific Interior (frontier wave; spread during glaciation); (2) Pacific Hinterland (spread to Pacific late in glaciation, chronology of spread to America unknown), (3) Pacific Rim (late glacial to postglacial); (4) Chukchi-Kamchatkan and Eskimo-Aluet families (spreads from *ca.* 5000 BP). The first three strata are not discrete in reality.

Guinea, while the Pacific Rim province is limited to New Guinea. Australia and New Guinea were sundered by the postglacial sea-level rise, a process which began about 16,000 years ago, was substantially complete 11,000 years ago, and was fully complete 8000 years ago when the remaining land bridge was flooded. The Pacific Rim province in Australasia must have formed after Australia and New Guinea had begun to separate, as it is lacking in Australia but well represented in New Guinea; but probably not long thereafter, as this province is an intensified late phase of the Hinterland province, which does appear in northern coastal Australia. Thus the formation of the Australasian Pacific Rim province may have begun with movements of seafarers to northwestern coastal New Guinea as early as 16,000 years ago. The last immigrations belonging to this province were colonizations of northern coastal New Guinea by Austronesian speakers beginning 4000 years ago; the spread of Austronesian languages through Melanesia and out into the Pacific continued until recent times (for Austronesian see *e.g.*, Ross 1988; Pawley & Ross 1993; Kirch 1996). The Austronesian family dispersed about 6000 years ago from the vicinity of Taiwan and spread, in occasional colonization episodes rather than a continuous stream, over insular Southeast Asia to reach Melanesia and New Guinea some two millennia later. Though the early Austronesians carried agriculture and their predecessors probably did not, other aspects of the history of its spread may well be typical of what must have occurred from time to time in the 12,000 years from the formation of the Pacific Rim province in Australasia to the arrival of Austronesians in New Guinea (and indeed of the history of overseas colonization in Melanesia and Australasia for the last 50,000 years). Importantly for the present argument, the Austronesian languages in New Guinea are still mostly coastal and exhibit some of the Pacific Rim features (verb-initial word order, numeral classifiers, *m* in second person pronouns).

The relative chronology of entries of the earlier strata must be as follows. The Interior province formed first, as a result of early colonizations, and the Pacific Hinterland province formed later and perhaps not greatly earlier than the Pacific Rim province. More time probably elapsed between the Interior and Hinterland entries than between the Pacific Hinterland and Pacific Rim strata. An absolute chronology for the earlier strata is less certain. The Pacific Hinterland is most clearly visible in northern Australia near where the postglacial sea-level rise first cut off Australia from New Guinea beginning about 16,000 years ago; thus this stratum is older than 16,000 years, but (in view of its clarity) probably not greatly older.

The stock half-life calculation presented above provides several different ways of estimating an age for the Pacific Rim population of languages. The crudest way is to count the number of stocks in the population and compute the age of the group in the event that it is a single genetic grouping (derived from a single entrant to the Americas or New Guinea, or a single Siberian or Southeast Asian dispersant). In my sample the number of language stocks in the American Pacific areas (Alaska-Oregon, California, Mesoamerica, and western South America) is 44, and there are proposals for deeper genetic connections which, if proven, would reduce the number to 39 or less. The age of such a group would be 48,000 years — much too early for any plausible entry to the Americas, let alone a relatively late entry. Of course, it is quite likely that some of the languages in the Pacific Rim zone survive from earlier entries and spreads and do not belong to the Pacific Rim population but happen to share their territory. Reducing the size of the population by one-quarter to one-half to accommodate this possibility yields ages of 42,000 and 36,000 years, still much earlier than any archeological evidence of habitation and implausibly early for a relatively recent entry. These results indicate that the Pacific Rim population of America is not a single genetic lineage, since all consequences of assuming deep genetic unity are implausible, but they do not tell us the age or the actual number of genetic lineages.

Personal pronoun systems with *n* in the first person singular and *m* in the second person singular are one of the markers of the Pacific Rim group. Since personal pronouns are easily inherited and not often borrowed, let us hypothesize that the languages with *n : m* pronouns may be ancient sisters and compute the age of their hypothetical family. (Recall, though, that the *n : m* paradigm is not a sufficient genetic marker. Relatedness of all the *n : m* languages can be hypothesized but not assumed.) The languages with *n : m* pronouns in the western Americas represent from 12 to 17 stocks (depending on exactly where the Pacific Rim boundary is placed, and on whether some possible but unproven deep groupings are taken to be stocks). This points to an age of 30,000 to 36,000 years, again too early for these stocks to be descendants of a single entrant to the Americas (given that the Pacific Rim population is a relatively recent formation), although not implausibly early for an ancestor in Siberia or northern Asia.

The conclusion to be drawn from these various calculations is that the Pacific Rim population is highly unlikely to be a set of sister languages descending from a single immigrant into the Americas. The signature historical markers that cluster in this population must result from a mixture of inheritance and acquisition (from substratum or borrowing). Let us now consider the ages for two proposed but unproven deep groupings within the population: the Hokan and Penutian groups centered in California and Oregon. The Hokan group (see Langdon and Jacobsen 1996; Kaufman 1988) contains most or all of Karok, Chimariko, Shasta, the Achomawi-Atsugewi family, Washo, Yana, the Pomoan family, Salinan, the Yuman-Cochimi family, Seri, and the Tequistlatec-Jiqaque family (listed from north to south as they run from northern California to southern Mexico), and perhaps Esselen and/or Chumashan of coastal California, a total of about 12 branches. Each branch is an isolate or small family, and as relatedness between any of them has not been demonstrated each can be regarded as its own stock. Then the age of the family — if it is a family — is on the order of 30,000 years.

Penutian consists of a dozen families for which some further subgrouping is usually posited: The Miwok-Costanoan and Yokuts families of central California; Maiduan of northern California and Klamath-Modoc, Sahaptian, and Molala of Oregon; Wintun of northern California and Coos, Siuslawan, and Alsean of coastal Oregon, and Takelma-Kalapuyan and Chinookan also of Oregon (this subgrouping from Callaghan 1997; DeLancey & Golla 1997; Golla 1997; see also Goddard 1996). If each of these four groupings were a stock — and this has not been proven — then Penutian would be 12,000 years old. Without these intermediate groupings it would be of the same age as Hokan, since both groups contain about a dozen stocks.

Thus, if both Hokan and Penutian are genetic groups, then the age of the Pacific Rim population (which includes them) is such as to accommodate the dispersals of two ancient families, one perhaps 12,000 years old and one probably older. These were separate events which occurred within the larger, and therefore presumably still older, Pacific Rim population. By this metric too, the age of the Pacific Rim population is greater than the firm archeological age for settlement of the Americas.

The Pacific Rim province in New Guinea contains — depending on how certain questions of classification are resolved and exactly where its inland boundary is placed — some 15-20 stocks. If they all descend from a single ancestor, the age of the set is 30,000 to 36,000 years. Descent from a single ancestor, however, is implausible: Austronesian is one of these stocks, it is known to have originated from abroad,

TABLE 5. Combined immigration and diversification. A constant stock diversification rate of 1.5 is assumed. Age = age of the population. Rate = period (in years) within which there is an average of one surviving linguistic colonization. Numbers of stocks rounded to whole numbers.

Age	Rate	Number stocks
12,000	2000	10
	4000	6
16,000	2000	14
	4000	8
20,000	2000	21
	4000	11

and its history is probably typical. A combination of the regular branching rate and an average immigration rate will give an approximate age for a set of stocks derived by a combination of immigration and subsequent diversification. Table 5 shows some figures for various colonization rates.

New Guinea has been colonized by languages from different branches of the Eastern Malayo-Polynesian branch: by Oceanic languages in the east and by others in the west. This amounts to colonization by one stock (Austronesian) in approximately 4000 years (the age of the Eastern Malayo-Polynesian branch). Though it is admittedly risky to base a model on a single example, it can at least be concluded that a colonization rate of one stock immigrant in 4000 years is plausible. On the other hand, the Austronesian immigration also shows that independent entries could occur in two regions: The west (where colonizations came from Halmahera) and the east (where they came from New Britain and New Ireland). The early Austronesians introduced agriculture where they spread, and agriculture can lower stock densities. Therefore, while today the Melanesian islands to both the west and the northeast of New Guinea are almost entirely Austronesian-speaking, in pre-Austronesian times stock diversity was probably greater, so colonizations at those two entry points might have come from entirely different families. Hence two immigrations per 4000 years, or one per 2000, may be a better estimate of the pre-Austronesian rate.

Table 5 shows that, for the 2000-year immigration rate, an age of 16,000 years for the province is expected. Of course, some minority of the languages in the province must descend from earlier immigrants, so the number of stocks originating in the Pacific Rim colonization phase must be fewer than the 15–20 actually in the province — perhaps 12–15. Assuming that one-quarter of the stocks are earlier survivors lowers the age of the province, though it is still probably older than 12,000 years. Though this measure is highly approximate, it yields an age for the Australasian Pacific Rim province that is reasonably consistent with the date of 16,000 years or less computed above based on the postglacial sea-level rise.

To summarize this survey of language origins and language spreading around the Pacific Rim, the presence of the same three strata in the Americas and Australasia suggest that a single southeast Asian source fed the growing linguistic populations of both areas as languages moved out into the Pacific and others moved north to Siberia and thence to Alaska. Initially, when the spread began, the structural typology of the source area seems not to have differed greatly from that of the rest of the world (which, at that time and for modern human languages, was the Eurasian tropics and Africa). Hence the Interior Province areas belong structurally in the western Old

World (Table 4). But then a very distinctive structural type made itself felt and created the second and third strata, giving rise to the markers of the Pacific Rim population. The Pacific Rim colonization thrust reached Australasia perhaps as early as 16,000 years ago and was active until recent times when it produced Austronesian colonizations. It reached the Americas (spreading coastally in Asia up to Beringia and then down the American Pacific coast) sufficiently long ago to have formed a large and diverse population stretching the entire length of North and South America by about 5000 years ago when the interior Siberian linguistic type, represented by Eskimo-Aleut, severed Pacific Rim linguistic continuity. The internal age of the Pacific Rim province in the Americas is great: To derive its total of over 40 stocks from regular diversification and immigration (with a single entry point and a 2000-year periodicity, and assuming 10 of those stocks are remnants of the earlier population) would take 24,000 years, and to derive them from a single ancestor would take even longer.

Conclusion

The calculations given here have indicated that modern human language is over 130,000 years old if monogenetic and over 100,000 years old if polygenetic with 10 separate ancestors; both figures are highly approximate minima. Considerations of paleodemography and linguistic geography support polygenesis. Languages (and modern humans) spread out of the original small range to extend from Africa to southeast Asia, and the eastern edge of this range contributed the initial colonizing languages to Australasia (colonized overwater from mainland Asia, with coastal landfalls) and also the Americas (colonized overland via Beringia, probably coastally). When this colonization began — over 50,000 years ago on archeological evidence from Australia — there was a gradual west-to-east clinal distribution of structural features in languages. Occasional additional colonizations continued on both fronts, and the combination of immigration and divergence created the tremendous linguistic diversity of New Guinea and the Americas. A datable linguistic event is the appearance of the Pacific Rim structural type in the east Asian staging area for both colonization fronts. That type must have begun spreading out in both directions some 20,000 years ago and perhaps earlier. It reached Australasia about 12,000–16,000 years ago, with the waning of the glaciers, and has continued to spread, colonize, and recolonize in insular southeast Asia, Melanesia, and Oceania. It reached the Americas at some undetermined time (early, though relatively late in the settlement history of the Americas) and continued occasional immigration until, with the Eskimo-Aleut spread about 5000 years ago, a very different structural type entered the pipeline. The origin of language was vastly earlier than the rise of the Pacific Rim type, but long-standing language spreading in various directions from Asia has given that type impact on half of the areas in the sample used here.

This brief survey shows that nongenealogical comparison can tell us a good deal about when and where modern language arose and about the proximate and ultimate major geographical contributors to large populations of languages. Far from constituting an obstacle to reconstructing language origins, the fade-out point of about 6000 years for tracing linguistic descent makes it possible to design a uniform sample, determine sizes of linguistic populations, compute genetic density on a consistent basis, estimate an average rate of divergence through branching, and estimate rates of linguistic immigration. These in turn have made it possible to identify and date some salient phases in the origin and dispersal of the world's languages. On the most realistic estimates, modern language as we know it is at least as old as modern humanity. Its origin was not a single point on a map or a single event in time, but a gradual process that unfolded in several different speech communities of varying degrees of discreteness. A continuous history from that origin to the present day can be traced in the spreads of originally local developments, of which this paper has described the main developments around the Pacific.

Endnotes

[1]In linguistics, genetic refers to classification by descent, or cladistic analysis. It is not literally genetic, since linguistic descent does not involve genes. Linguistic descent and biological descent are completely independent of each other, in that every individual carries the genes of his or her ancestors but by no means everyone speaks the language of their ancestors. This is self-evidently true for a large immigrant nation like the United States and for languages of the colonial period, but it is more common in other societies than is generally recognized by non-linguists. The French, for instance, carry genes inherited from the Gauls but speak a descendant of the language of the Romans. The Bulgarians carry, at least in some part, the genes of the Bulgar Turks who entered the Balkan peninsula in the eighth century, but they speak the Slavic language which the Bulgars soon thereafter took over from their neighbors. Language shift — the process where a society or speech community shifts, usually over the course of a few generations, to another language ¾ is common in societies of all types and sizes. In fact the number of speech communities whose languages go back in unbroken inheritance, without shifts, for more than a few millennia is probably small.

[2]Comparing more than two languages can reduce the number of resemblants needed to demonstrate nonchance resemblance — provided a significant number of the languages compared participate in each putative cognate set. Threshold numbers are given in Nichols (1997) (*e.g.*, each set of putative cognates with generic resemblances must occur in at least 4 out of 6 languages compared, or 5 out of 10, or 15 out of 50). To my knowledge these criteria have never actually been reached in multiple (or mass) comparisons; every multiple comparison I have seen offers too few attestations per cognate, and/or too loosely defined resemblances, for the results to be considered nonchance.

[3]A *bottleneck* is any substantial reduction in the number of continuing descent lines, as occurs in colonization, where only a few of the world's individuals or languages enter the new land to proliferate. The entering population is the *founder* or *founding population*, and *founder effects* occur when the inheritable traits of the founders show up among the descendants not in their expected or worldwide frequencies but in unusual frequencies reflecting their accidental idiosyncratic frequency in the founding population.

[4]Using generic consonants is more appropriate, as we need to match Wiyot *kh* to Algonquian *k,* and the Yurok glottalization to nonglottalization in the other branches. The overall probability of the whole paradigm, using the 0.07 probability for the generic consonants, is $0.07 \times 0.07 \times 0.07 \times 0.07 \times 0.25 \times 0.25 \times 0.25 \times 0.25 = 0.000000094$, about nine in a hundred million or one in ten million.

[5]In the earlier work on Algic, both Sapir and Haas realized the importance of the pronominals but apparently believed that cognate vocabulary and regular sound correspondences were also an essential ingredient in the proof. As Goddard (1975) shows, the pronominals are sufficient evidence and working out cognates and correspondences are secondary to demonstrating relatedness, no matter what Sapir and Haas may have believed about what they were doing.

[6]The firm initial branches are: Anatolian, Tocharian, Celtic, Armenian, Greek, Albanian, Italic, Germanic, Balto-Slavic, Indo-Iranian. (Of these, Anatolian and Tocharian are now extinct.) Poorly attested ancient Indo-European languages such as Phrygian, Thracian, and Illyrian may or may not be separate branches.

[7]For these computations I have taken the traditionally inhabited world to be what it was during the last glaciation, subtracting the area under glaciers and adding an estimate of the exposed continental shelf from southeast Asia to Australia-New Guinea, where the exposed shelf is likely to have been well populated.

[8]Two caveats are in order. First, both comparative work and description in New Guinea are just beginning; comparative work may reduce the number of stocks, but on the other hand field work continues to turn up new families and isolates. If description can possibly keep up with extinction in New Guinea, it is possible that in some ten to twenty years we will have a different number of stocks for New Guinea, but at present it appears likely that newly discovered stocks will cancel out newly discovered genetic connections. Second, the initial branching rate of stocks in New Guinea, as in high-diversity zones generally, is low. Lower branching rates yield higher linguistic ages.

[9]The literature on the modern human dispersal is vast. Recent overviews include Howell (1996), White (1996).

[10]An overview is found in Howell (1996). Harpending *et al.* (1993), Sherry *et al.* (1994), Relethford and Harpending (1995) posit a population bottleneck and a reduction to perhaps only a few thousand individuals, followed by population growth during the global expansion. This reduction followed the evolution of modern humans, and the reduced population had several subgroups, of which the largest is now best represented in sub-Saharan African populations.

[11]If as suggested in Note 10 about half of the population formed a single gene pool in the south, the size of the pool — a thousand to a few thousand individuals — suggests several languages while its biological genetic unity suggests much intermarriage and hence multilingualism and convergence. Migration frequencies estimated for the other populations by Harpending, Sherry, Rogers, and Stoneking. are far less than what is required for multilingualism and linguistic convergence, hence these ethnicities may have been more discrete.

[12]The bottleneck discussed in Notes 10 and 11 would have reduced the diversity but would still have left very different genetic lineages and structural types at distant parts of the range. It could easily have removed individual languages and lower branches while leaving most of the higher-level families with at least some representation on Earth.

[13]The rank-sorting of areas was either ascending or descending so as to put one or another bellwether area in the top half of the ranking. The choice of bellwether area has relatively little impact on the outcome. In the counts reported in Nichols (1997d), Africa was used as the bellwether area.

[14]Numeral classifiers are particles or affixes that are mandatory in phrases with numerals; the particular classifier used depends on the quantified noun, and classifiers often form elaborate shape-classified sets. Possessive classification is the analog, in head-marking languages, to declension classes in languages like the classical Indo-European ones. Declension classes are sets of case and/or number allomorphs, lexically determined by the noun and more or less orthogonal to gender and other classifications. Possessive classification is allomorphic sets of person-number possessive affixes, lexically determined by the possessed noun. It is rare and incompletely surveyed (for the semantics of the classes see Croft 1994), but appears to have a strictly Pacific Rim distribution.

Literature Cited

Austerlitz, R. 1980. Language-family density in North America and Eurasia. *Ural-Altaische Jahrbücher* 52:1–10.

Bender, M.L. 1969. Chance CVC correspondences in unrelated languages. *Language* 45:519–536.

———. Upside-down Afrasian. *Afrikanistische Arbeitspapiere* 50:19–34.

————. 1975. *Omotic: A New Afroasiatic Language Family.* (University Museum Series, 3.) Southern Illinois University, Carbondale.

Birdsell, J.B. 1953. Some environmental and cultural factors influencing the structuring of Australian Aboriginal populations. *Amer. Nat.* 87:171–207.

————. 1957. Some population problems involving Pleistocene man. *Cold Spring Harbor Symp. Quant. Biol.* 22:47–70.

Callaghan, C.A. 1997. Evidence for Yok-Utian. *Intl. Jour. Aner. Ling.* 63:18–64.

Croft, William. 1994. Semantic universals in classifier systems. *Word* 45:145–171.

DeLancey, S. & V. Golla. 1997. The Penutian hypothesis: retrospect and prospect. *Intl. Jour. Amer. Ling.* 63:171–202.

Diakonoff, I.M. 1988. *Afrasian Languages.* Nauka, Moscow, Russia.

Durie, M. & M.D. Ross, eds. 1996. *The Comparative Method Reviewed: Regularity and Irregularity in Language Change.* Oxford University Press, New York.

Ehret, C. 1995. *Reconstructing Proto-Afroasiatic (Proto-Afrasian): Vowels, Tone, Consonants, and vocabulary.* (University of California Publications in Linguistics 126.) University of California Press, Berkeley.

Embleton, S. 1986. *Statistics in Historical Linguistics.* Brockmeyer, Bochum, Germany.

————. 1991. Mathematical methods of genetic classification. Pages 365–388 *in* S. M. Lamb, & E.D. Mitchekk, eds., *Sprung from Some Common Source: Investigations into the Prehistory of Languages.* Stanford University Press, Stanford.

Fortescue, M. 1998. *Language Relations across the Bering Strait: Reappraising the Archeological and Linguistic Data.* Cassell Academic, London, U.K.

Goddard, I. 1975. Algonquin, Wiyot, and Yurok: Proving a distant genetic relationship. Pages 249–62 *in* M. D. Kinkade, K. L. Hale, & O. Werner, eds., *Linguistics and Anthropology: In Honor of C. F. Voegelin.* de Ridder, Lisse, The Netherlands.

————. 1996. The classification of the native languages of North America. Page 290 *in* Ives Goddard, ed. *Handbook of North American Indians, vol. 17: Languages.* Smithsonian Institution, Washington, DC.

Golla, V. 1997. The Alsea-Wintuan connection. *Intl. Jour. Amer. Ling.* 63:157–70.

Greenberg, J.H. 1960. An Afro-Asiatic pattern of gender and number agreement. *Jour. Amer. Orien. Soc.* 80:317–21.

————. 1963. *The Languages of Africa.* Indiana University Press, Bloomington.

Haas, M.R. 1958. Algonkian-Ritwan: the end of a controversy. *Intl. Jour. Amer. Ling.* 24:159–73.

Harpending, H. C., S. T. Sherry, A. R. Rogers, & M. Stoneking. 1993. The genetic structure of ancient human populations. *Curr. Anthropol.* 34:483–96.

Heath, J. 1978. *Linguistic Diffusion in Arnhem Land.* Australian Institute of Aboriginal Studies, Canberra, Australia.

Howell, F.C. 1996. Thoughts on the study and interpretation of the human fossil record. Pages 1–39 *in* W. E. Meikle, F. C. Howell, & N. G. Jablonski, eds., *Contemporary Issues in Human Evolution,* California Academy of Sciences Memoir 21. California Academy of Sciences, San Francisco.

Kaufman, T. 1988. A research program for reconstructing Proto-Hokan: First groupings. Pages 50–168 *in* S. DeLancey, ed., *Papers from the Hokan-Penutian Language Workshop, 1988.* Department of Linguistics, University of Oregon, Eugene.

Kirch, P.V. 1996. *The Lapita Peoples: Ancestors of the Oceanic World.* Blackwell, Cambridge.

Krauss, M.E. 1988. Pages 144–51 *in* W. W. Fitzhugh & A. Crowell, ed., *Many tongues — Ancient Tales. Crossroads of Continents: Cultures of Siberia and Alaska.* Smithsonian Institution, Washington, D.C.

Lamb, S.M., & E.D. Mitchell, eds. 1991. *Sprung from Some Common Source: Investigations into the Prehistory of Languages.* Stanford University Press, Stanford.

Langdon, M. & W.H. Jacobsen, Jr. 1996. Pages 129–130 *in* V. Golla, ed., Report on the Special Hokan Session in Albuquerque, July 1995. *Proceedings of the Hokan-Penutian Workshop, July 8–9, 1994 and July 5–6, 1995.* (Survey of California and Other Indian Languages, Report 9.) Survey of California and Other Indian Languages, University of California, Berkeley.

Mace, R. & M. Pagel. 1995. A latitudinal gradient in the density of human languages in North America. *Proc. R. Soc. Lond.* B 261:117–21.

Newman, P. 1980. *The Classification of Chadic within Afroasiatic.* Universitaire Pers, Leiden, The Netherlands.

Nichols, J. 1990. Linguistic diversity and the first settlement of the New World. *Language* 66:475–521.

———. 1992. *Linguistic Diversity in Space and Time.* University of Chicago Press, Chicago.

———. 1995a. The spread of language around the Pacific Rim. *Evol. Anthropol.* 3:206–15.

———. 1995b. Diachronically stable structural features. Pages 337–356 *in* H. Andersen, ed., *Historical Linguistics 1993. Papers from the Eleventh International Conference on Historical Linguistics.* John Benjamins, Amsterdam-Philadelphia.

———. 1996. *The comparative method as heuristic.* Pages 39–71 *in* M. Durie & M.D. Ross, eds., *The Comparative Method Reviewed: Regularity and Irregularity in Language Change.* Oxford University Press, New York.

———. 1997a. Modeling ancient population structures and movement in linguistics. *Annual Rev. Anthropol.* 26:359–84.

———. 1997b. Sprung from two common sources: Sahul as a linguistic area. *Archaeology and Linguistics: Global Perspectives on Ancient Australia,* P. McConvell & N. D. Evans, eds. Oxford University Press, Melbourne, Australia.

———. 1997c. The geography of language origins. Pages 267–278 *in Proceedings of the 22nd Annual Meeting.* Berkeley Linguistics Society, Berkeley.

———. (submitted) Of needles and haystacks: Searches and heuristics in comparative method. MS under review.

Nichols, J. & D.A. Peterson. 1996. The Amerind personal pronouns. *Language* 72:336–71.

Orel, V. & O. Stolbova. 1995. *Hamito-Semitic Etymological Dictionary.* Brill, Leiden, The Netherlands.

Oswalt, R.L. 1991. A method for assessing distant linguistic relationships. Pages 389–404 *in* S.M. Lamb & E.D. Mitchell, eds., *Sprung from Some Common Source: Investigations into the Prehistory of Languages.* Stanford University Press, Stanford..

Pawley, A. & M.D. Ross. 1993. Austronesian historical linguistics and culture history. *Ann. Rev. Anthropol.* 22:425–59.

Relethford, J.H. & H.C. Harpending. 1995. Ancient differences in population size can mimic a recent African origin of modern humans. *Curr. Anthropol.* 36:667–76.

Ringe, D.A., Jr. 1992. On calculating the factor of chance in language comparison. *Trans. Amer. Philos. Soc.* No. 82.

Roberts, R.G., R. Jones, & M.A. Smith. 1990. Thermoluminescence dating of a 50,000–year-old human occupation site in northern Australia. *Nature* 345:153–56.

Roberts, R.G. & R. Jones. 1994. Luminescence dating of sediments: new light on the human colonization of Australia. *Austral. Abor. Stud.* 1994:2–17.

Ross, M.D. 1988. *Proto Oceanic and the Austronesian Languages of Western Melanesia.* (Pacific Linguistics C-98.) Department of Linguistics, Research School of Pacific Studies, Australian National University, Canberra, Australia.

————. 1996. Contact-induced change and the comparative method: cases from Papua New Guinea. Pages 180–217 *in* M. Durie & M.D. Ross, eds., *The Comparative Method Reviewed: Regularity and Irregularity in Language Change.* Oxford University Press, New York.

Sapir, E. 1913. Wiyot and Yurok, Algonkin languages of California. *Amer. Anthropol.* 15:617–46.

Sherr, S.T., A.R. Rogers, H. Harpending, H. Soodyall, T. Jenkins, & M. Stoneking. 1994. Mis-match distributions of mtDNA reveal recent human population expansions. *Hum. Biol.* 66:761–5.

Thomason, S.G. & T. Kaufman. 1988. *Language Contact, Creolization, and Genetic Linguistics.* University of California Press, Berkeley.

Trask, R.L. 1996. *Historical Linguistics.* Arnold, London, U.K.

Woodbury, A.C. 1984. Eskimo and Aleut languages. Pages 49–63 *in* W. C. Sturtevant, ed., *Handbook of North American Indians, vol. 5: Arctic.* Smithsonian Institution, Washington, DC.

White, J.P. 1996. Paleolithic colonization in Sahul land. Pages 303–308 *in* T. Akazawa & E.J. E. Szathmáry, eds., *Prehistoric Mongoloid Dispersals.* Oxford University Press, Oxford, U.K.

The Origins of World Linguistic Diversity: An Archaeological Perspective

Colin Renfrew
The McDonald Institute for Archaeological Research
Downing Street
Cambridge CB2 3DZ, UK

The potential convergence of historical linguistics, prehistoric archaeology and molecular genetics offers hope of a new synthesis, in which the events and processes underlying the geographical distribution of human diversity. and specifically linguistic diversity, may be clarified. One would hope and perhaps imagine that the archaeological record would also be informative about the early emergence of linguistic ability as a specifically human attribute, and in particular about the time and context when a well-developed capacity for language first emerged. But so far the relationships between material culture and linguistic ability have proved difficult to establish. Early aspects of hominid diversity, such as the differing distributions of handaxe and pebble-tool cultures in earlier Paleolithic times, should be noted, as well as the very limited distribution of 'naturalistic' cave art and mobiliary art in Upper Paleolithic times. These are instances of geographical variability, for which linguistic correlates might conceivably be claimed. It is argued, however, that the most significant process underlying the 'spread zone' versus 'residual zone' pattern evident in the modern geographical distribution of language families was agricultural dispersal, with a time depth no greater than about ten thousand years.

It is suggested that population history is the factor common to the three potentially converging disciplines, and that recent and ongoing developments in molecular genetics are likely soon to clarify some outstanding questions.

At first sight the languages of the world today can teach us little about the origins of language, or even about the origins of linguistic diversity. The diversity is certainly there: It is estimated that there are some 6,000 different languages spoken in the world today. But the time depth is lacking. We have no direct knowledge of any language prior to the invention of writing in the Near East and then Egypt some 5,000 years ago, and then in China some 3,500 years ago, and then more widely from 3,000 years ago.

Fortunately, however, the languages of today contain much information relevant to their own histories. The resemblances or affinities between two languages, in terms

The Origin and Diversification of Language
Editors, N.G. Jablonski & L.C. Aiello

Memoirs of the California Academy of Sciences
Number 24, Copyright ©1998

of their phonology, morphology and vocabulary, can indicate very clearly that they are related. The discipline of historical linguistics uses such insights in a systematic way to group such related languages into what may be termed 'language families.' Like the taxonomies of biology, such classifications may go beyond arranging like with like in terms of superficial appearance (phonetic classification). In certain circumstances they may reasonably allow inferences about family relationships, suggesting that some branches are more closely related than others, and permit inferences about hypothetical ancestors. Such inferences may allow the emergence of a pattern which reflects the historical process of descent: A genetic classification.

For over a century archaeologists and historical linguists have struggled to use the archaeological data for the human occupation of the continents of the Earth to give some insights into the formation of these language families. At times scholars have confused linguistic groups with supposed racial groups, and in the earlier half of this century notions of racial supremacy brought about an unhappy episode both in the historical sciences and in world history. But today it should be possible to avoid such fallacious equations. It is necessary also to avoid simplistic assumptions about how languages change, and indeed about how 'peoples' move.

It is my belief that a new synthesis is today possible, using three disciplines which are in a sense formally independent, since they use different classes of data: historical linguistics, prehistoric archaeology and molecular genetics. Modern linguistics is today increasingly taking a worldwide view, studying the whole wide range of languages, and not focusing to the exclusion of others upon the languages of Europe and Western Asia. From this global view new insights are emerging.

Molecular genetics, as applied to living human populations, is now the fastest growing field of study about the human past. For just as the languages of the world today contain information about their own past, so do the genes within human populations. Studies of nuclear and mitochondrial DNA are allowing the similarities and differences between individuals and between groups to be studied, and, as in the linguistic case, phonetic classifications may in favorable cases lead to genetic classifications (Figure 1).

There is , moreover, the hope that the recovery of ancient DNA from preserved human remains may give direct information about the genetic composition of individu-

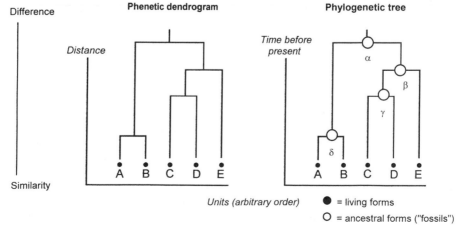

FIGURE 1. The potential isomorphism between phonetic dendrogram and genetic descent.

als long dead, which will offer a control and a test on the genetic inferences which have been based upon the study of living materials.

Prehistoric archaeologists are thinking in new ways about culture change and culture process, and models of change are being constructed which are more appropriate to our understanding of early cultural dynamics. Moreover archaeology offers a much better grasp upon time depth than do the other two disciplines which join with it in the new synthesis. Radiometric dating methods do now reliably allow the provision of reasonably accurate dates, in calendar years, for the deposits and the artifacts which the archaeologist discovers.

In reality it is not easy to bring together these three different classes of data: the linguistic, the molecular genetic and the archaeological. There is perhaps a tendency in each discipline to favor its own data set, and, it has to be said, to draw preferentially upon the other disciplines to support current inferences, in such a way that the argument often becomes a circular one. Certainly it cannot be too firmly asserted that languages in themselves tell us nothing about the genetic composition of their speakers, and genes carry no direct linguistic implications: There are, in practice, strong correlations, but (as I shall hope to emphasize) these arise from historical contingencies, not from any general equivalence between languages and genes.

The first central point which I wish to make is that there was in fact only one historical reality. People lived upon the face of the Earth: Specific languages were spoken at particular times at definite places. Those people had genetic compositions of specific kinds, and to the extent that their descendants survive, those DNA patterns albeit transformed and modified, survive to influence and indeed determine the DNA of those descendants. Those same people had settlements and used tools, and exploited plants and animals, and remains of all these things persist in the archaeological record to this day.

The new synthesis will not come about until all three classes of data are used with respect. Most archaeologists of my acquaintance are very hazy indeed about the patterns visible when one studies language families, or nuclear and mitochondrial DNA. Most molecular geneticists are prone to make hasty conclusions not only about the population histories which might have given rise to the genetic patterns which they observe, but also about possible linguistic or archaeological correlations. I have to say that I have found rather few historical linguists who are willing to recognize the archaeological or molecular genetic data at all: One sometimes has the impression that languages are supposed to evolve and change of their own accord without any human agency.

Nowhere are these shortcoming, these failures in bringing different classes of data to bear, more evident than in the matter of chronology, of dating. Archaeologists, as I have said, do have sure dating methods, but they are used for dating artifacts, and artifacts in themselves tell us nothing of language or of genes. Molecular geneticists use a variety of frameworks of inference for estimating genetic rates of change, and there is no doubt that these are continually being refined. But it is sometimes difficult to escape the conclusion that the foundations are insecure. The recent suggestion by Pääbo (1996) that estimated mutation rates for mitochondrial DNA may have been up to an order of magnitude in error certainly gives cause for reflection.

But if molecular genetics have problems with dates (or rates) these are as nothing compared to those of the historical linguist. Most historical linguists today reject the techniques of "glottochronology" as formulated by the Swedish (which assumed an approximately constant rate of word loss in all languages at all times).

But while few linguists will go so far as Joseph Greenberg in developing an alternative formulation (defining a core vocabulary, and assuming an exponential rather than a linear decay process), many still find it possible to offer approximate dates for the formation or dispersal of this or that protolanguage. Some of these rely upon the archaeology for the dating of vocabulary features — and many are the pitfalls which I could catalogue in the supposed dating of the 'wheel' or the 'horse' in Indo-European studies, from Gustav Kossinna to Jared Diamond. But some historical linguists make the claim that they operate by principles of dating which go beyond those of glotto-chronology or of linguistic paleontology. I have never been able to discover what these principles are, and have always suspected that they depend upon circular reasoning. The only effective solution must be the bringing into proper perspective of the genetic, the linguistic and the archaeological data, and that is no easy task.

Today I would like to indicate the growing body of evidence that suggests that there is indeed some meaningful patterning in the distribution of the world's language families. I shall seek to suggest that there are indications, which we can recognize, of language groupings which have been in place geographically for well over ten thousand years, before the end of the last ice age, the termination of the Pleistocene period. These languages and families would therefore document the conclusion of the dispersal of our own species, *Homo sapiens sapiens*, during the Pleistocene period. And I would like to indicate that there are other more recent patterns which we can recognize, many of them associated with the inception of farming, and then the widespread radiation of agricultural and farming technologies, which began to take place some 10,000 years ago. There is a growing body of archaeological evidence which can be brought to bear upon these matters. But what makes the current situation so interesting is that there is a considerable flow of data from molecular genetics which bears very strongly upon these hypotheses. It can tell us nothing about early language directly, as noted above. But it can tell us a great deal about population history. It is indeed the concept of population history that lies at the heart of the new synthesis, since it is of direct relevance in each of the three intersecting fields with which we are dealing (Figure 2). In each case it is the processes of inference, the models of change, that require further scrutiny.

The Origins of Cultural Diversity and the Question of Language Origins

When did linguistic competence develop among our ancestors? Here I should first like to draw attention to some of the limitations of the view of language origins that are currently so widely held. Although it is in many ways plausible that there should be a correlation between the emergence of anatomically modern humans, of new aspects of material culture (such as the blade industries of northern Europe, first seen at the onset of the Upper Paleolithic) and the development of full speech capacity, there is in fact little concrete evidence that such was the case. There are, moreover, earlier indications of regional diversity in the archaeological record which should certainly be noted, even if linguistic correlates are not proposed for them.

At first sight, indeed, the pattern of world linguistic diversity today casts little light upon that deep and challenging question of the origins of language. I had almost become resigned, at symposia on early language, to being the man at the end: The one who deals with the past ten or twenty millennia. This may seem a formidable time depth to the conventional historical linguist. But with the assumption, almost univer-

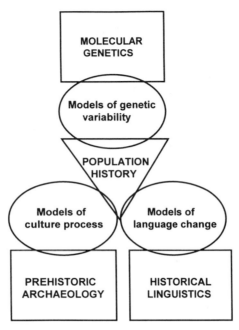

FIGURE 2. The intersecting fields of the new synthesis.

sally held, that all human groups were anatomically modern by at least 40,000 years ago, and all speaking fully developed languages at that time, by the time I would have anything to offer, the process of initial language formation, that is to say the development of linguistic ability is already complete. To put the matter in more colloquial terms, it is all over bar the shouting.

But I have recently come to feel that some of the widely accepted conclusions about the early history of language are not so well established as they might seem. The data are inevitably few, and some aspects of the archaeological record which do show some degree of coherent patterning are perhaps being undervalued.

Today many archaeologists, geneticists and linguists accept what I should like to call the "Michelangelo effect." They accept that anatomically modern humans appeared in Europe some 40,000 years ago. They accept, quite rightly, that all anatomically modern humans today (and of course we all are) have fully developed linguistic capacities, which are therefore to be taken as characteristic of *Homo sapiens sapiens.* And they note that the transition from Middle to Upper Paleolithic industries in the archaeological record at that time show the emergence of new tool forms, notably blade industries, and worked bone and antler, indicative of the skills associated with the new species. Add to this the wonderful appearance of cave art in France and Spain only some 5,000 years later, and you have a "package" which, with the eye of faith, can be seen to constitute a single "Human Revolution" scarcely less miraculous than the Creation of Adam.

The prominent exponents of this view, such as Lewis Binford or Paul Mellars are critical, skeptical about the abilities of the Neanderthals who preceded our own species, questioning, for instance, the alleged evidence for deliberate burial in Middle Paleolithic times. Sometimes I wonder if we are not in face of some miraculous new "Creation," and that wonderful image from the Sistine Chapel ceiling comes into my mind. By the "Michelangelo effect," then, I mean the assertion that there was a revolutionary emergence at one and the same time of anatomically modern humans, of full linguistic capacities, of the ability to think conceptually, of a much wider range of social and cultural behaviors (manifested in new lithic industries and soon in cave art).

But as these scholars are well aware, the emergence of anatomically modern humans took place much earlier, presumably in Africa around 150,000 years ago, and is seen already in southwestern Asia at the Qafzeh Cave around 100,000 years ago.

Here I want to draw your attention to just two interesting questions. First the ability to conceptualize. And second the matter of regional diversity. Each has been taken by some scholars as an indication of linguistic ability. But both are clearly evident in the archaeological record of the Middle Paleolithic period, hundreds of thousands of years before the emergence of modern humans and of the widely assumed development along with them of advanced linguistic capacities

The Handaxe

For some time scholars have debated the significance of those striking core tools, called 'handaxes' (Figure 3), which are found over a time range of at least half a million years in Africa, western Asia and Europe, the characteristic product of our immediate prehuman ancestor, *Homo erectus*. Although some scholars, such as Davidson and Noble (1993) have regarded them as simply worked-out cores, the byproduct of the manufacture of flake tools, most have taken the view that these are deliberately made tools (*e.g.*, Toth & Schick 1993).

I have recently been impressed by the arguments of the philosopher John Searle (1995) that many of the most important foundations of our social life are what he terms "institutional facts," conceptual formulations by which society functions (such

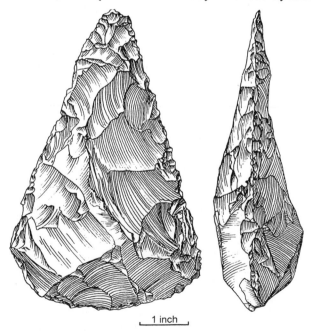

1 inch

FIGURE 3. Handaxe from site of Swanscombe, Kent. Based on Oakley (1967:72).

as rank, power, gender (as opposed to sex), value, wealth, money, *etc.*) They require human institutions for their existence, and indeed institutions of a kind which we would normally assume to require the cognitive capacities of modern humans. These may be contrasted with 'brute facts,' often facts of nature, which exist quite independently of language or of any other institution. They are not dependent upon linguistic conventions or on the fairly sophisticated tacit understandings and conventions among individuals that form the basis for our social lives. It may certainly be argued that the archaeological record can give unequivocal indications of 'institutional facts' and of the concepts associated with them: The stone cubes of the Indus Valley civilization around 2000 BC as indicative of modular systems of weighing and of counting are a case in point (Renfrew 1982).

What is interesting here, however, is that Searle very clearly associates what he terms 'agentive functions' — seen for instance in the production of a specific artifact form designed to fulfill a particular purpose — with such institutional facts. He gives the example of a screwdriver, stressing the distinction between features which are intrinsic to nature and others which are relative to the intentionally of observer, users, *etc.* But I would argue that in this case what is good for the screwdriver is good also for the handaxe, so long as we are willing both to recognize it ourselves as a distinctive tool type and also to infer or assume that its makers also saw it in that way, as a purposive product not just the unintended consequence of making flakes.

Such analyses are helpful. They help to show us that we are dealing here with well-defined concepts. But we should remember, as Thomas Wynn reminds us (Wynn 1993), that this need not necessarily imply the existence of a spoken language. Merlin Donald in his *Origins of the Modern Mind* (Donald 1991) regards the era of *Homo erectus* as the mimetic phase of hominid cognitive evolution, preceding the mythic phase (with its stress on language) of early *Homo sapiens sapiens*. And Bloch (1991) has reminded us that culture is not necessarily linguistic. We should note the importance of imitation, or serial memorization, in so much mimetic learning. This point is well made in a diagram by David Clarke (1968) (Figure 4).

We see here that no speech is needed for one individual to teach another how to make a handaxe, nor indeed would speech be needed to teach how to use it. Speech is not needed to show a young child how to sit on a chair, and the concept "chair" does not need the verbal formulation of the word "chair" for its understanding and communication. To say this is simply to make a general remark about the understanding and communication of agentive functions.

This point can be used in two diametrically different ways. Those scholars who see a long and slow evolution of language as likely, will argue that vocal utterance is likely to have accompanied the formulation of the concept (*e.g.*, of the handaxe) and its practical embodiment through manufacture. They will take it that vocal means will have been found already in the Lower Paleolithic period to accompany such 'institutional facts.' They will argue that there will already have been signs, and perhaps sounds (or 'words') indicative of 'handaxe' or of 'fire' (when that came to be produced deliberately). These can be regarded, within the perspective developed by Searle, as conceptual formulations of a kind which many of us would imagine require a degree of cognitive sophistication difficult to achieve without the use of language.

An alternative view is that the Lower and Middle Paleolithic do indeed represent a 'mimetic' phase, and that the production of well-defined tool forms does not require any very sophisticated conceptualizing power. Moreover such conceptualization as was needed need not have been language dependent. The real breakthrough will have

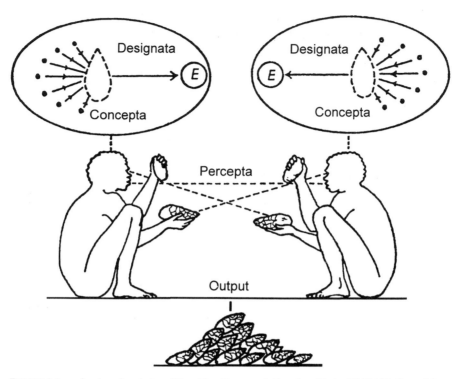

FIGURE 4. Learning by mimesis (possibly without language). Based on Clarke (1968:182, figure 39).

come with the formation of developed linguistic powers, perhaps 40,000 years ago and that these were exclusively restricted to our own species.

Regional Diversity

Regional diversity in behavior within a single species must be regarded as cultural behavior — that is to say learned behavior passed on locally within a regional tradition — if it does not have a genetic origin (which would imply regional diversity in the genome). For that reason local cultural traditions have excited the attention of archaeologists as displaying an aspect of behavior which is particularly characteristic of humans, although it is true that some other species do show patterns of regionally specific learned behavior. It seems to be the case, however, that some aspects of regional diversity seen in the Paleolithic period have not received sufficient consideration: They too may have a bearing upon the emergence of developed linguistic ability.

It may be that when we speak in global terms of the Pleistocene and refer to Neanderthals or to 'Upper Paleolithic humans' we are making the same category error of dealing in gross and unrefined categories which today we are ready to criticize when we read anthropological works of a century ago which speak of 'primitive man' or 'primitive art.' It may be this global generalization which has obscured some of the significant regional variation in the archaeological record. It is seen already in the Lower Paleolithic, and some aspects persist right through into the Holocene period, so that there are features here which could conceivably have a bearing upon our understanding of quite recent linguistic diversity.

One of the earliest known instances of regional diversity is the disparity which existed around half a million years ago, following the dispersal out of Africa of *Homo erectus*, in the distribution of lithic artifacts. We have already spoken of the handaxes which are such a frequent feature of the Lower Paleolithic of western Europe, and of the same period in Africa. It is notable, however, that in southeast Asia, where remains of the same hominid species are found, and in some other areas including Eastern Europe, there are no handaxes. Instead we find the 'pebble tool tradition' which in fact resembles in some ways the lithic industries found in Africa during the earlier, pre-*erectus* period, and generally attributed to that earlier ancestor *Homo habilis* (Figure 5).

It is particularly interesting that this same regional divide continues right up into the Upper Paleolithic period, and indeed in southeast Asia even later, where the Hoabhinian lithic tradition is found. Blade industries which we associate with the European Upper Paleolithic are not a universal feature. Although I am myself persuaded by the genetic evidence for an out-of-Africa origin for our own species, it has to be said that the 'multiregional' hypothesis, with a local hominid evolution from *erectus* to *sapiens* would sit more easily with the above interpretation of the lithic sequence. Presumably the analysis has to be undertaken at a much finer level before it can bear such weighty constructions. But the point here is that there are regional diversities in culture that must have an important place in the evolutionary history. If this long-standing differentiation does not have a genetic origin (and few would suggest that the tendency to make handaxes rather than pebble tools is genetically determined) does it not reflect a long-standing cultural tradition which might also be of linguistic significance?

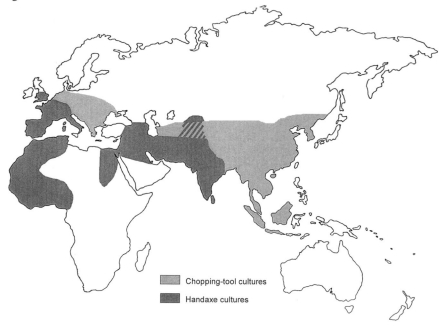

FIGURE 5. Map of handaxe *vs*. pebble industries: spatially distinct traditions of tool making, both associ - ated with *Homo erectus* about 1 million to 100,000 years ago. Based on Burenhult (1993:64).

The second case of regional localization which deserves emphasis is that of cave art. The casual reader might have the impression that the remarkable painted caves of France and Spain have their counterparts over much of the world. Did we not learn recently, and it is indeed a remarkable discovery, that there is rock art in Australia going back some 40,000 years and perhaps more, and that there may be an unbroken tradition of rock art in that subcontinent from that time until the present?

A closer analysis will, however, distinguish between the Franco-Cantabrian cave art and the rock shelter art which is indeed a very widespread feature globally, but indicative of more recent hunter-gatherers and perhaps of pastoralists. In the first place the Franco-Cantabrian cave art is not (as we know it) a rock shelter art: It is found deep in limestone caverns which are difficult of access now and were difficult of access then. And in the second place there is a coherent style in the Aurignancian and Magdalenian art of France and Spain which deserves to be defined closely in a way that avoids such terms as 'naturalistic' or 'figurative,' but yet which indicates how these images differ in the impressions which they give from those of most rock art styles. In short they are different. This was a special phase in a limited region which began 35,000 years ago, and is without known parallel elsewhere. The point is emphasized for us by the 'Venus' figurines and other carvings associated with the Gravettian culture in much the same area, but with an eastward extension to Siberia (Figure 6). These again are, I believe, without parallel for the Paleolithic period. There is no virtue in our basing our discussions about early language on the assumption that the human abilities which produced these visual symbols were universally available to our species from 40,000 years ago onwards.

Once again we have a notable case of regional diversity, this time in the display (in the archaeological record) of the outstanding conceptual abilities implicit in the production of Franco-Cantabrian cave art and in the small Gravettian sculptures. Such

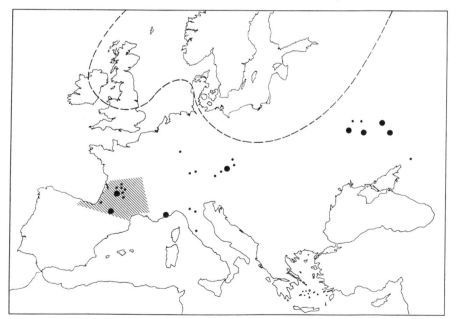

FIGURE 6. The distributions of Franco-Cantabrian cave art (hatched area) and Gravettian "Venus" figu - rines which are restricted to Europe *ca*. 29,000-22,000 years ago.

abilities cannot, however, be claimed as a universal feature of our species in the Upper Paleolithic period: Their documentation is very restricted geographically. Did these evident conceptual abilities have no linguistic counterpart? Might not this imply some degree of linguistic diversity?

Linguistic and Cultural Evolution

In discussing the 'Sapient Paradox' (Renfrew 1996b), that is to say, the disparity between the assumed fully human status (anatomically and linguistically) of our species by some 100,000 to 80,000 years ago, and the considerable delay before we see anything very remarkable in its behavior, I suggested that in our analysis we should indeed lay more stress on *praxis*, on actual activity and behavior, and upon the artifacts which document it and which often motivated it.

Biologists are used to speaking, among living species, of the genotype (defined by the genes) and the phenotype (reflecting the living organism). But in human affairs it is the 'prototype,' representing the actual behavior, which interests us, rather than the physical form with all its potential for interesting behavior but perhaps with little to show for it.

I begin to feel that we should not assume modern or complex behavior until we have proof of it. That is why the discussion of the limited distribution of rupestrian and mobiliary art is so illuminating. These were not human universals in the Upper Paleolithic, but very restricted in their scope.

How long did it take language to evolve? Let us imagine that there is a gene or related set of genes which govern the capacity for complex linguistic behavior: Such an assumption is indeed made among nearly all evolutionary biologists. Whether or not we embrace the "Michelangelo effect" we can recognize that fully modern linguistic ability, common to all living human groups, represents a significant mutation or series of mutations from what went before. Let us further imagine that this mutation or set of mutations occurred in a given local area and restricted time period. It is widely believed today that enhanced linguistic facility would confer adaptive advantage, and that the gene would diffuse successfully through the population. But the interesting question is: What happens next?

Language is a social phenomenon: It is spoken between people. It implies not only a shared vocabulary, but shared understandings and concepts, shared 'institutional facts.' When and how did these arise, and how long did that take? Should we expect to see behavioral correlates in the archaeological record?

At first sight we might imagine that these new, gifted individuals in the population would soon be forging their own language. It might at first be a 'private' language, like that shared by the Bronte siblings, but it would soon become public. The insight that it might grow among siblings and cousins is probably right, since it would be these individuals who would share the new genetic endowment. But the Bronte parallel may not be a sound one. It is one thing to imitate what is already done in a different way: Quite another to originate *ab initio*. The extensive literature on 'stimulus diffusion' reminds us that it is easier to reinvent the wheel, when you have seen it, than to invent it in the first instance.

Do we, in those special cases where symbols were being used with particular richness and profusion, as with the Gravettian figures of 20,000 years ago, and the Franco-Cantabrian paintings from 35,000 years ago, see cases where conceptual and symbolic virtuosity may be reflecting the development of new symbolic skills in oral and hence verbal communication as well as visual communication — *i.e.*, language skills?

The point which I am making here is that we should not make the mistake of assuming that the behavior of hunter-gatherers in recent years is a sound guide to that of the hunter-gatherers of 30,000 years ago. The former have the benefit of the same length of time of cultural and social evolution as do farmers and city-dwellers. Indeed is it to be concluded that, over the past 40,000 years, there has been continuing selection of those individuals who are linguistically able, and against those with less developed linguistic capacities?

There may be a significant distinction to be drawn between the genetic mutations (genotypic) which led to linguistic *capacity* or *ability* (phenotypic) on the one hand, and the actual achievement, through the evolutionary development and use of language on the other hand (praktotypic) of those linguistic skills which we associate with the exponents of all known languages. Whether the indigenous Tasmanians, who at the time of their encounter with Europeans were accounted to have the most impoverished known material culture among hunter-gatherers, had the same sophisticated language skills which we associate with surviving hunter-gatherers is unfortunately a question which history has left unanswered.

The Language Farming Dispersal Hypothesis

It is appropriate now to change the focus of discussion from the question of the origins of linguistic ability to that of the origins of linguistic diversity or capacity. Of course one would expect the latter to be related to, indeed dependent upon, the former. But many linguists would hold that it is not practicable to undertake linguistic reconstructions beyond a time depth of some five or six thousand years.

They would argue that the processes of linguistic divergence (including word replacement and loss) operate in such a way that a language at one time point will have been so transformed over the millennia in the course of evolution and transmission to its daughter languages that no trace of the parent will be evident through the study of the offspring. The existence of such a linguistic time barrier of five or six thousand years is currently coming under question. But caution is still appropriate and it may still be appropriate to refrain at this time from linking questions of the origins of language (as a human capacity) with those of the origins of languages (as reflected in contemporary linguistic diversity).

Several linguists have remarked on the marked difference in the nature of the geographical distribution of language families. Austerlitz (1980) has contrasted patterns of language-family density, and Nichols (1992) made the useful distinction between what she terms linguistic 'spread zones' and 'residual zones.'

When a language family displays the 'spread zone' pattern it displays what the linguist may term a low genetic density (*i.e.*, a limited number of linguistic units unrelated by descent from a common language ancestor) over a sizable area, and a relatively shallow time depth. The 'residual zone' pattern shows more language families, greater linguistic diversity within the language family, and greater antiquity of the linguistic stocks there. The Caucasus is a good example of a 'residual zone,' and is sometimes regarded as a linguistic refugium.

Here I wish to reiterate the hypothesis, already formulated in rather different form (Renfrew 1992, 1996a) that most of the world's language families which show a 'spread zone' distribution are the result of a process of farming dispersal. The same point has been persuasively developed by Peter Bellwood in a number of influential papers (*e.g.,* Bellwood 1996).

It would seem that the distinction is a fundamental one, which has also a chronological significance. All the "residual zone" language distributions have been in place for at least 10,000 years, since before the end of the last glaciation (Class A in Table 1). The early settlement dates now available for Australia and for New Guinea (*i.e.,* the 'Indo-Pacific' languages) explain their place in category I. It should be noted, however, that only the North Australian languages show the characteristics of a 'residual zone': For reasons as yet not well understood the remaining languages of Australia (the so-called Pama-Nyungan group) show the characteristics of a 'spread zone.'

All the "spread zone" distributions are the product of dispersals within the past 10,000 years (Class B in Table 1). The most significant cases, those listed in category II are indeed farming dispersals. But the role of northern climate-sensitive adjustments by hunter-gatherers after 10,000 BP should be noted (category III) and of course that of long distance maritime colonization over the past five centuries (category V). Only in a very few cases is it appropriate to ascribe the distribution of an entire language family to the process of "élite dominance" (category IV). This may however be the effective mechanism for much of the later distribution of the Altaic language family (made possible by the development of horse riding), as well as for the Indo-Iranian branch of the Indo-European family.

It should be noted that in the table some language families are indicated within single quotes: This is intended to indicate that by many linguists they are not regarded as true language families (in the linguistically genetic sense of sharing a common origin from an ancestral protolanguage). They may instead simply represent language areas where previously unrelated languages have come to share a number of characteris-

TABLE 1. "Residual Zone" (Class A) and "Spread Zone" (Class B) Language Families (Renfrew 1996a, with modifications).

The present distribution of each language area is accounted for by one of the following five processes:

CLASS A: PLEISTOCENE

I.   *Initial colonization prior to 12,000 BP:*
     'Khoisan', 'Nilo-Saharan' (plus later 'aquatic' expansion), Northern Caucasian, South Caucasian, "Indo-Pacific" (plus later farming changes), North Australian, 'Amerind.' Localised ancestral groups of II and III (below)

CLASS B: POST-PLEISTOCENE

II. *Farming dispersal after 10,000 BP:*
     Niger-Kordofanian (specifically the Bantu languages), Afroasiatic, Indo-European, Elamo-Dravidian, Early Altaic, Sino-Tibetan, Austronesian, Austroasiatic.

III. *Northern, climate-sensitive adjustments after 10,000 BP:*
     Uralic-Yukaghir, Chukchi-Kamchatkan, Na-Dene, Eskimo-Aleut

IV. Élite dominance:
     Indo-Iranian, Later Altaic, Southern Sino-Tibetan (Han)

V   *Long-distance maritime colonization since 1400 AD:*
     Mainly Indo-European (English, Spanish, Portuguese, French).

tics. It should be noted that all of these, like the others in category I show the 'residual zone' pattern.

In earlier discussions of farming dispersal I have emphasized the demographic effects of the spread of farming, and have emphasized the "demic diffusion" model initially proposed by Ammerman and Cavalli-Sforza. It is indeed the case that many farming economies have been propagated through the gradual expansion of the farming population, and this point has on a number of occasions been very well argued by Bellwood (*e.g.*, 1996). However it is appropriate also to recognize the point made by Zvelebil (1996) and others, that the techniques of farming may well be taken up by the indigenous hunter-gatherer population. In such a case one might well have farming transmitted, but without a significant degree of gene flow, or of language replacement.

It is, however, worth developing what one might term the "substitution model" for language replacement in the wake of farming dispersal. Here one may draw upon the model developed by Zvelebil (1996:325) but with a rather different purpose (Figure 7).

Zvelebil here envisages a three-phase availability model for the transition to farming, where the indigenous population acquires the new domesticates and the techniques of the farming economy, while itself remaining genetically little altered. Rhret (1988) has, however, described a situation such as this where the local group, formerly hunter-gatherers, take up the language of the farmers along with their economy and technology, while retaining their own ethnic and more particularly genetic identity. The process of acculturation which Zvelebil envisages allows time for many elements of the speech of the farmers to be acquired along with the necessary technology. This then would be a case of language replacement, although the case is very different from that of demic diffusion, and there is plenty of room for features of the indigenous language, whether lexical or morphological, to survive in the new language which the indigenous inhabitants adopt, or rather form by their adoption of so much of the farmers' speech and technology. In such cases, where the new speech is acquired by substitution rather than by demic diffusion, we should expect the newly-emerging language family to show more diversity, and to owe more to the language being replaced (which would form a more evident substrate) than in the demic diffusion case.

There are many instances of language families whose distribution may be assigned to a language-farming dispersal process, whether by colonization (demic diffusion) or by acculturation (substitution). A number of them have been conveniently listed by Bellwood (1996:469) (Table 2).

Bellwood, in a number of articles, has very persuasively dealt with the Austronesian languages. The case of the Niger-Kofdofanian languages (notably the Bantu languages) has been well set out by a number of authors including Phillipson (1977). In a number of papers I have suggested that the source for the farming dispersal which carried the Indo-Euuroean protolanguage to Europe was the Anatolian lobe of the southwestern Asian zone of agricultural origins. The northeastern lobe, towards Turkmenia, may well have transmitted farming techniques to the region where the proto-Altaic languages were spoken, which later gave raise to the Altaic expansion. The southwestern lobe was the starting point for the Elamo-Dravidian languages. And it has always seemed to me that the only coherent process underlying the Afroasiatic linguistic unity must be the dispersal of sheep and goats, and later cereals, from the Jordan-Palestine area across to North Africa, although the story there may be a long and complicated one.

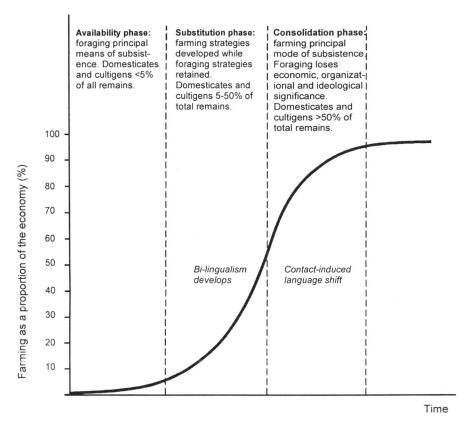

Availability phase: foraging principal means of subsistence. Domesticates and cultigens <5% of all remains.

Substitution phase: farming strategies developed while foraging strategies retained. Domesticates and cultigens 5-50% of total remains.

Consolidation phase: farming principal mode of subsistence. Foraging loses economic, organizational and ideological significance. Domesticates and cultigens >50% of total remains.

Farming as a proportion of the economy (%)

Bi-lingualism develops

Contact-induced language shift

Time

FIGURE 7. Linguistic adjacency acceptance: The adoption by hunter-gatherers of the language of neighboring cultivators through conduct-induced language shift. Based on Zvelebil (1996: 325), with additions.

Glover and Higham (1996) have recently reconsidered the origins of rice cultivation in southeast and east Asia considering the possibility that rice cultivation began first on the Assam/Yunnan border area, from which agriculturists expanded down the Yangtze River, reaching the early farming site of Hemudu by 5000 BC and standing at the head of the proto-Austro-Tai linguistic grouping. Movement from the nuclear area westwards via the Brahmaputra River into eastern India would have brought the Proto-Munda languages. Southward expansion down the Mekong River would have been responsible for the dispersal of Proto-Mon-Khmer, and down the Red River for Proto-Viet. These conclusions are at present hypothetical, but they do associate the early dispersal of rice cultivation with several language families of southeast Asia.

The effects of the development of farming in New Guinea was significant enough for that island, but the economy did not in this case prove an expansive one, partly perhaps because it was associated with highland areas. For that reason it is in many ways appropriate to see upland New Guinea as a 'residual zone.' Farming there is not the product of some dispersal process, but an indigenous development.

In the case of the Americas there were indeed more localized dispersal processes underlying the distributions of the language families indicated in Table 2. But there were no continent-wide effects, mainly because the relevant plant domesticates (there

TABLE 2. Regions of early agricultural development and farming dispersals (based on Bellwood 1996).

Region of early agriculture	Associated language families
sub-Saharan Africa	Niger-Kordofanian
Southwest Asia	Elamo-Dravidian
	Indo-European
	Altaic
	Afro-Asiatic
China (north)	Sino-Tibetan
China (south)	Austroasiatic
	Austronesian
	Tai
	Hmong-Mien (Miao-Yao)
New Guinea	Many Papuan families
Mexico	Otomanguean
	Uto-Azteccan
	Mayan
	Mixe-Zoque
Andes/Upper Amazon	Chibchan/Paezan
	Qhechua/Aymara
	Arawakan
	Panoan

being few animals) were not so economically decisive as the cereal crops of southwestern Asia had been in that continent, and were indeed still to prove to be in the Americas once transported thither by the European colonists.

This discussion may be consolidated into some three hypotheses:

Hypothesis 1. Most language families of 'spread zone' type are the product and result of farming dispersals.

Hypothesis 2. Most farming dispersals had clearly identifiable linguistic concomitants, often resulting in language families of 'spread zone' type.

Hypothesis 3. Most linguistic configurations of 'residual zone' type are the products of initial population dispersals into previously uninhabited territories, taking place (apart from those in the northern periarctic zone) prior to 10,000 BP.

As I see the position, from the standpoint of the hoped-for synthesis heralded above, this approach has the strength that it recognizes that linguistic replacement generally takes place in pace with some degree of population replacement, or at the least in situations of marked technical change and acculturation. Languages do not change of their own accord in some purely linguistic dimension: Linguistic change is a social phenomenon, with appropriate social and economic correlates which, in favorable cases, should be visible in the archaeological record.

The Genetic Dimension

One of the great reasons for optimism about the new synthesis is that there is a steady flow of genetic data which may ultimately serve to resolve some outstanding controversies. As noted earlier, there is no expectation of any immediate correlation between genetic and linguistic data. Attempts to equate trees of genetic descent with those of notional linguistic evolution are to a large extent misleading. This is partly because the pace of linguistic evolution is so much greater than genetic. But in particular it overlooks the historical dimension. Had there been no major episodes of language replacement, mainly powered by farming dispersals, most of the world's language families might well be of 'residual zone' type, having been in position for tens of thousands of years. There might then be case for comparing genetic with linguistic affinity. In reality, however, the genetic map, like the linguistic, has been radically modified by these dispersal processes. So indeed there is certainly a strong correlation between the language family of a particular ethnic group and its genetic composition, but that is because both are the product of replacement in relatively recent times, as the result of a dispersal process.

This point may be illustrated effectively by the work of Excoffier and his colleagues, using classical genetic markers, in their examination of African ethnic groups, classified by language family (see Renfrew 1992b:464). They examined the frequency of the different gamma globulin alleles in a number of African sampling populations which were chosen on a tribal (*i.e.*, in effect a linguistic) basis. When they classified these in terms of similarity and difference (by producing a phonetic dendrogram of the kind seen in Figure 1) it turned out that the classification achieved by looking at the genetic markers in fact grouped together the Afroasiatic speaking tribes, the Niger-Kordofanian speaking tribes, *etc.* In other words, the genetic characteristics (as determined from the blood samples) were a good predictor of linguistic affinity also.

Molecular genetics may well be in a position to support or contradict a number of the hypotheses set out above. For as I stressed at the outset, the common ground between the three disciplines of historical linguistics, molecular genetics and prehistoric archaeology is population history. But the interpretive frameworks are not yet fully developed in molecular genetics, nor, as noted earlier, are mutation rates yet well established.

To give an example of the changing fortunes of molecular genetic arguments it may be interesting to compare various results relating to the language farming hypothesis for Europe. In previous papers I have argued that the early dissemination of the Proto-Indo-European language in Europe was the product of a farming dispersal of the type discussed above, with Anatolia (the northwestern lobe of the southwestern Asiatic nuclear farming area) as the starting point. An earlier proposal to account for the spread of the Indo-European languages was the mounted warrior horseman hypothesis — the suggestion that the proto-Indo-European language originated in what is now the Ukraine and was carried westwards in the fourth millennium BC in a military conquest activated by the early domestication in that region of the horse. This still has its adherents, but its standing has diminished recently with the realization that claims for the early domestication of the horse have been exaggerated, and with the confirmation that horse riding for military purposes came to Europe only after the introduction of the horse and chariot, not long before 1000 BC (Renfrew, in press).

One of the earliest investigations of the genetic background to the demic diffusion hypothesis for the origins of farming in Europe was offered by Cavalli-Sforza and his colleagues (1993), who undertook a principal components analysis of classical genetic markers among living populations of Europe. The first principal component (representing 28% of the variability) showed clear clines from southeast to northwest. This was interpreted by them as giving clear indications of the demic diffusion process accompanying the dispersal of agriculture (Figure 8).

188   RENFREW

This did not necessarily support the language-farming hypothesis, since it was
still possible that the dispersal of Proto-Indo-European could be a later event, but it
was nonetheless taken as support for the importance of the farming dispersal phenomenon itself.

A statistical analysis using analogous genetic data for North Africa and other areas
of Eurasia beyond Europe (Barbujani *et al.* 1994) produced comparable results for
Europe and the Near East and (less confidently) for North Africa, thus supporting the
importance of farming dispersals in southwestern Asia and thus, it was argued, to the
language-farming hypothesis.

An interesting study using data from mitochondrial DNA of living populations in
Europe, recently undertaken by Richards, Sykes and their colleagues (1996) led to
the identification of a number of mitochondrial lineages (Figure 9). Estimated divergence times for these suggested that most of them could be dated back into the Upper
Paleolithic period. It was concluded that the population composition of Europe was
largely constituted at this early date, and that, while later arrivals could be recognized
in the data, these were of relatively minor importance.

It was, however, a weakness of the study by Richards and his colleagues that they
did not have mtDNA samples from eastern Europe, and few from Anatolia. For if the
mitochondrial DNA lineages of Anatolia around 7000 BC were already much like

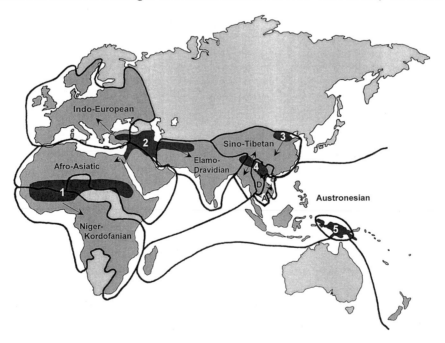

FIGURE 8. Major areas of primary domestication of selected principal food plants and distribu tions of selected language families whose extent is here ascribed to agricultural dispersal. The ar eas of primary crop
domestication are numbered: 1-sorghum/millet; 2-wheat/barley; 3-millet; 4-Asian rice; 5-taro/sweet po -
tato. Southeast Asian language families indicated by letters are D-Daic; A-Austroasiatic. (Note: the Indo-
European and Elamo-Dravidian distributions reflect the hypothetical agricultural dispersals and do not
show the subsequent spread of the Indo-Iranian languages. The agricultural dispersal underlying the Aus -
tronesian family distribution is believed to have originated in southeast Asia but was based subsequently
on yam, taro and tree fruits).

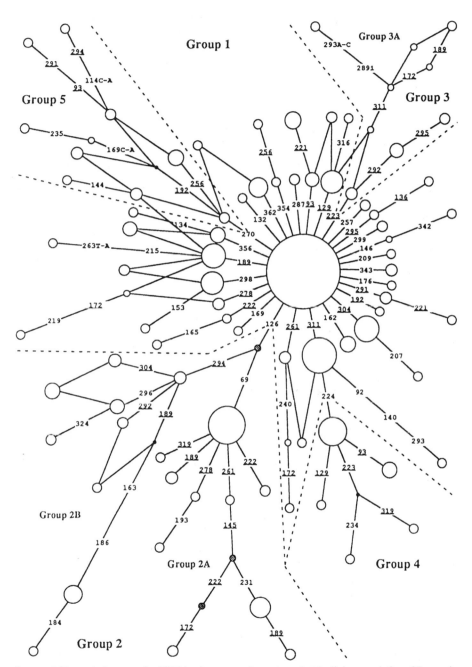

FIGURE 9. Network diagram of mtDNA haplotypes used to suggest that the living population of Europe is mainly of Paleolithic origin although it is suggested that group 2a is descended from Neolithic immigrants (based on Richards *et al.* 1996:192).

those of Europe, even a significant demic diffusion process might not show up strongly in the genetic composition of modern populations. As Comas and his colleagues (1996) remark, following a study of mtDNA and the population history of Turkey in relation to Upper Paleolithic and Neolithic dispersals,

> It is intrinsically difficult to separate the genetic effects of these two diachronic waves, which had very similar geographic origins and expansion paths. However it is possible that the reduced population size during the Upper Paleolithic allowed drift to act deeply on gene frequencies but had little effect on sequence diversity, as it is likely that the European population did not suffer any narrow bottleneck. In this case, the effect of the expansion of farming (that is, a sharp increase in mobility and population size) on gene frequencies could have been deep, transforming a random variation pattern into a cline, but would have had few consequences on mtDNA sequence diversity, which would reflect more ancient events (p. 1076).

The interpretive story does not end there, however. For recently Haeseler, Sajantila and Pääbo (1996; see also Watson *et al.* 1996) have emphasized a different approach to the genetic data, which lays more emphasis upon the history of whole populations rather than just of individual lineages. They stress that the study of pair wise sequence distributions (in mitochondrial DNA from recent populations under study) can illuminate population history. They show that different patterns are to be observed in groups which at an earlier time have expanded notably in size (as a result of agricultural expansion) in comparison with those whose size has remained constant over time, as is the case with hunter-gatherers. Pääbo (1996) has gone further and suggested that the mutation rate between different regions of the mitochondrial DNA is variable, and may have been underestimated. In this case the divergence times estimated by Richards and his colleagues would be serious overestimates, and the patterning in their data might after all be consistent with the demic diffusion model for agricultural dispersal in Europe.

I have set out these various approaches to the problem because I think that they give a very clear idea of the dynamism of the current situation. Within a few years that situation will have become very much clearer, and the genetic evidence will have made a very significant contribution, as it is already beginning to do, to our understanding of population history. I do not doubt that this will also have significant implications for historical linguistics, as indeed it will for prehistoric archaeology.

Conclusion

In the preceding section I have sought to indicate that the application of molecular genetics, which has only recently been brought effectively to bear upon some of these issues, is likely to transform our understanding of human population history. If it does we can expect to learn much more about the operation of various social processes, such as human migration, population replacement or demic diffusion, which are directly relevant to language history. In particular the language-farming hypothesis, that a significant component of modern language diversity may be explained as the consequence of farming dispersals, may be open to testing. Our picture of the origins of modern world linguistic diversity is likely to develop rapidly over the next decade or so.

Whether there will be comparable progress in the question of the much earlier origins of language as a general attribute of our species is more doubtful. There are grounds for optimism that molecular genetics will indeed contribute further to our understanding of the early history of human evolution. But no secure framework of inference has yet been constructed such as would permit one to infer the capacity for language from material culture, or indeed from the fossil remains of our early ancestors. In consequence the patterns of very early cultural diversity discussed in the first part of this paper may continue to tantalize us without offering any secure grounds for identifying or dating the emergence of speech by means of the archaeological record.

Literature Cited

Austerlitz, R. 1980. Language family density in North America and Eurasia *Ural-Altaisches Jahrbucher* 52:1–10.

Barbujani, G., A. Pilastro, S. de Domenico, & C. Renfrew. 1994. Genetic variation in North Africa and Eurasia: Neolithic demic diffusion vs. Paleolithic colonization. *Amer. Jour. Phys. Anthropol.* 95:137–54.

Bellwood, P. 1996. The origins and spread of agriculture in the Indo-Pacific region: Gradualism and diffusion or revolution and colonization. Pages 465–498 *in* D.R. Harris, ed., *The Origins and Spread of Agriculture and Pastoralism in Eurasia* UCL Press, London, U.K.

Bloch, M. 1991. Language, anthropology and cognitive science. *Man* 26:183–98.

Burenhult, G. 1993. *The First Humans*. Harper Collins, New York.

Cavalli-Sforza, L.L., P. Menozzi, & A. Piazza. 1993. Demic expansion and human evolution. *Science* 259:639–646.

Clarke, D.L. 1968. *Analytical Archaeology*. Methuen, London, U.K.

Comas, D., F. Calafell, E. Mateu, L. Perez-Lezaun, & J. Bertranpetit. 1996. Geographic variation in human mitochondrial DNA control region sequence: the population history of Turkey and its relationship to the European populations, *Molec. Biol. Evol.* 13:1067–1077

Davidson I. & W. Noble. 1993, Tools and language in human evolution. Pages 363–388 *in* K.R. Gibson & T. Ingold, eds., *Tools, Language and Cognition in Human Evolution.* Cambridge University Press, Cambridge, U.K.

Donald, M. 1991. *Origins of the Modern Mind.* Harvard University Press, Cambridge.

Ehret, C. 1988. Language change and the material correlates of language and ethnic shift. *Antiquity* 62:564–573.

Glover, I. C. & C.F.W. Higham. 1996. New evidence for rice cultivation in south southeast and east Asia, Pages 413–441 *in* D.R. Harris, ed., *The Origins and Spread of Agriculture and Pastoralism in Eurasia*. UCL Press, London, U.K.

von Haeseler, A., A. Sajantila, & S. Pääbo. 1996. The genetical archaeology of the human genome. *Nature Genetics* 14:135–140.

Nichols, J. 1992. *Linguistic Diversity in Space and Time.* University of Chicago Press, Chicago.

Oakley, K.P. 1967. *Man the Tool-Maker*. British Museum (Natural History), London, U.K.

Pääbo, S. 1996. Mutational hot spots in the mitochondrial microcosm. *Amer. Jour. Hum. Genet.* 59:493–496.

Phillipson, D. W. 1977. The spread of the Bantu languages. *Sci. Amer.* 236:106–114.

Renfrew, C. 1982. *Towards an Archaeology of Mind*. Cambridge University Press, Cambridge, U.K.

————. 1992a. World languages and human dispersals: A minimalist view. Pages 11–68 *in* J.A. Hall & I.C. Garvie, eds., *Transition to Modernity: Essays on Power, Wealth and Belief.* Cambridge University Press, Cambridge, U.K.

————. 1992b Archaeology, genetics and linguistic diversity, *Man* 27:445–78.

———. 1996a. Language families and the spread of farming, Pages 70–92 *in* D.R. Harris, ed., *The Origins and Spread of Agriculture and Pastoralism in Eurasia.* UCL Press, London, U.K.

———. 1996b. The Sapient Paradox: How to test for potential. Pages 11–14 *in* P. Mellars & K. Gibson, eds., *Modeling the Early Human Mind.* McDonald Institute, Cambridge, U.K.

———. in press. All the King's Horses: Assessing cognitive maps in later prehistoric Europe, *in* S. Mithen, ed., forthcoming.

Richards, M., H. Corte-Real , P. Forster , V. Macaulay , H. Wilkinson-Herbots, A. Demaine , S. Papiha, R. Hedges , H.-J. Bandelt, & B. Sykes. 1996. Paleolithic and neolithic lineages in the European mitoochondrial gene pool *Amer. Jour. Hum. Genet.* 59:185–203.

Searle, J. 1995. *The Construction of Social Reality.* Allen Lane, Harmondsworth, U.K.

Toth N. & K. Schick. 1993. Early stone industries and inferences regarding language and cognition. Pages 346–362 *in* K.R. Gibson & T. Ingold, eds., *Tools, Language and Cognition in Human Evolution.* Cambridge University Press, Cambridge, U.K.

Watson E., K. Butler, R. Aman, G. Weiss, A. von Haeseler, & S. Pääbo. 1996. mtDNA sequence diversity in Africa. *Amer. Jour. Hum. Genet.* 59:437–444.

Wynn, T. 1993. Layers of thinking in tool behavior. Pages 389–406 *in* K.R. Gibson & T. Ingold, eds., *Tools, Language and Cognition in Human Evolution.* Cambridge University Press, Cambridge, U.K.

Zvelebil, M. 1996. The agricultural frontier and the transition to farming in the circum-Baltic region, Pages 323–345 *in* D.R. Harris, ed., *The Origins and Spread of Agriculture and Pastoralism in Eurasia.* UCL Press, London, U.K.

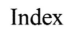

Index

Index

A

B